Accidental Cure

Extraordinary Medicine for Extraordinary Patients

Living Life By a Symphony of Strings and Meridians

Dr. Simon Yu, M.D.

Accidental Cure

Extraordinary Medicine for Extraordinary Patients

Living Life By a Symphony of Strings and Meridians

1st Edition

Prevention and Healing, Inc.

For information, address:
10908 Schuetz Road
St. Louis, Missouri 63146

www.preventionandhealing.com
www.accidentalcure.com

Printed in the United States of America

ISBN: 978-0-9797342-6-7

I dedicate my book to my grandmother, Anna Ko;
my father, Peter Hong Jun Yu;
my mother, Theresa So Wha Park Yu;
my wife, Jane Kate Yu;
my son, Louis Yu,
and to all my patients.

Acknowledgements

Many people have contributed to the creation of this book, and it is impossible to recognize and acknowledge everyone. I have been writing short educational articles for approximately 20 years; it could be said that the contacts, subjects, and knowledge base that I used to write those articles contributed to the publication of this book. The more articles I wrote, the more I wanted to publish a book. The patient success stories, in particular, seemed appropriate for a book's chapters. I am particularly grateful to one of my patients, Ed Mass. For many years, Ed has helped to prepare my short articles for *The Healthy Planet* magazine in St. Louis, and he also archived them on my web site (www.preventionandhealing.com).

I would like to thank Harvey Walker, M.D., Ph.D., who introduced me to the world of alternative/complementary medicine in St. Louis 20 years ago. The first two subjects were nutrition and chelation therapy. After meeting Harvey, there was no turning back to traditional internal medicine.

My enthusiasm for alternative medical conferences in the United States and Europe helped me find a path to energy medicine, and one of my most important contacts was Dr. Douglas Cook, D.D.S. His dental/medical conferences introduced me to the connection between dental problems and incurable medical conditions. He introduced me to the art of Acupuncture Meridian Assessment using an electroacupuncture according to Voll (EAV) device and taught me how to uncover hidden dental/medical conditions.

Learning how to use an EAV device is similar to learning how to play a violin. It's a big hurdle to master Acupuncture Meridian Assessment, just as it is to master the violin. As a first grader, I was forced to take violin lessons. Little wonder, as a young boy, I was determined to avoid an uncle who provided violin lessons, making me apply hours and hours of practice. As a physician, once I recognized the importance of EAV, I practiced and practiced and practiced, just as I had with a violin. I knew that if I persevered, eventually the practice would pay off—and it has!

Walter Sturm, Ph.D., from the Occidental Institute Research Foundation (OIRF) in Canada has provided meaninglful annual conference tours in Germany for exploring European biological medicine (as well as fine food, wine, and of course, beer). I appreciate the many private OIRF lectures that Walter has organized from the world's most well-respected scientists and biological medicine practitioners (including Professor Fritz Albert Popp, Ph.D.).

I am in debt to many pioneers in the field of alternative/complementary medicine, including Hulda Clark, Ph.D., N.D., Dietrich Klinghardt, M.D., Ph.D., Thomas Rau, M.D., George Goodheart, D.C., Garry Gordon, D.O., (H) M.D., Jim Clark, founder of Star Tech Health Services, and developer of the software/hardware for the electroacupuncture according to Voll (EAV) device as well as many other exceptional people.

Mary Jo Fahey has been instrumental as a book publishing consultant, coordinating and reorganizing my many scattered articles into a coherent book format. Her knowledge of nutrition and the field of alternative medicine has been outstanding, and her skills have enriched my writing, resulting in an orderly and reader-friendly book. I also appreciate Shawn Cornell's creative cover design, as well as Kay Urbant's keen eye as a copy editor and proofreader.

To all my patients who taught me how to be a physician in real lifetime situations and who encouraged me to explore the unknown in the field of medicine: after so many years of dealing with my EAV device, I'm certain that they would agree that it's best I did not choose to become a professional violinist.

Lastly, I could not write this book without my wife, Kate. She is always willing to proofread for me late at night and has been continuously supportive in so many ways.

Our Genes Are Not the Whole Symphony

Dr. Nihal S. DeSilva, M.Sc., Ph.D.

For many years, traditional medicine has been searching for genetic abnormalities that explain medical conditions. However, recent biomedical research provides many examples of medical conditions that appear to be shaped by additional factors, inexplicable by a DNA sequence variation alone. The result of this discrepancy has been growth in the field of "epigenetics." This term refers to the study of changes in gene expression without an underlying change in a DNA sequence.

Unlike genetic mutations, epigenetic changes are considered to be reversible, and nutrition is emerging as the most modifiable variable—implying that nutrients play a fundamental role in human cell physiology, our health, disease and what "epi" genetic characteristics are passed along to future generations (epi means "on top of" or "in addition to").

Thus, I find this excellent book, *Accidental Cure*, written by Dr. Simon Yu, M.D., very exciting as it opens an active investigation into the pathways of holistic medicine governed by epigenetics. The publication of this book by Dr. Yu is very timely, due to the recognition that epigenetic changes may be at the root cause of such diseases as cardiovascular disease, autism, cancer, diabetes, asthma, and several other significant illnesses.

Increased interest in epigenetic medicine has prompted the National Institutes of Health (NIH) to fund a "Roadmap Epigenomics Program" ($190 million). The NIH has defined the "epigenome" as chemical compounds that modify or mark the genome in a way that tells it what to do. These marks are not part of the DNA, but can be passed from cell to cell during cell division and from one generation to the next.

The information provided by Dr. Yu encompasses the miracle of natural healing, which is governed by the body's internal biocybernetic system. The internal biological terrain (epigenome) of the body is of paramount importance to health and disease. Dr. Yu's unique expertise is to make a critical assessment through the use of an Acupuncture Meridian Assessment (AMA) technique. The existence of various "acupoints" in the human body has been demonstrated by early Chinese medicine and is now accepted as an alternate method for diagnosis of health and disease. Dr. Yu, as a practicing physician with over 20 years of expertise in internal medicine, can discuss in great depth acupoint meridian changes in the human body caused by heavy metals, dental problems, parasite infestations, and food allergies. The use of the Acupuncture Meridian Assessment technique by Dr. Yu is a very effective way to monitor the status of the organ systems governed by the meridian system.

Dr. Yu has presented the underlying effects of agents that assault the human immune system. In a thorough manner, Dr. Yu presents a very valid and coherent view of whole-body epigenomics. The importance of food (nutrition) is discussed in a uniquely imaginative manner under "Food Crimes," "Food Remedies," and "Peak Performance Diet." A highly informative list of 81 "Boxed Topics" also provides the reader a wealth of supplemental information on the topics discussed in the various chapters of this book.

As a lecturer and biomedical researcher, I recommend this book to the general public and health care providers, especially physicians, nurses, dietitians, and medical researchers who are interested in optimum health and holistic medicine for the 21st century. Dr. Simon Yu has given us an authoritative, easy-to-read book, providing a solid background and solutions for understanding the various ramifications and problems we face in approaching preventive care via holistic medicine.

Nihal S. DeSilva, M.Sc., Ph.D.
Adjunct Professor (Nutrition & Immunology)
Washington University (Danforth Campus)
and BioGene, Inc.
St. Louis, Missouri

Table of Contents

Part I: Introduction

Chapter 1: Accidental Cure

Chapter 2: Biological Terrain and Biocybernetic Medicine

Chapter 3: Acupuncture Meridian Assessment (AMA)

Part 2: Staying Healthy in a Toxic World

Chapter 4: Heavy Metals

Chapter 5: Dental Death Trap

Chapter 6: Fighting the Body's Invaders: Parasites

Chapter 7: Parasites and EAV

Chapter 8: Food Crimes

Chapter 9: Food Remedies

Chapter 10: Peak Performance Diet

Part 3: My Articles

Chapter 11: Food-Related Articles

Chapter 12: Holistic Medical Articles

Chapter 13: Integrating Internal Medicine With Alternative/Complementary Medicine

Part 4: Patient Success Stories and Testimonials

Chapter 14: Conquering Cancer

Chapter 15: Solving Lung and Heart Problems

Chapter 16: Leaky Gut, Leaky Brain, Irritable Bowel, Irritable Mind

Chapter 17: Lazarus Effects (Nervous System– Related Problems)

Part 5: My Crock Pot Ideas

Chapter 18: Crock Pot Ideas?

Chapter 19: More Crock Pot Ideas

Part 6: Conclusion

Chapter 20: Time To Heal: New Medicine Based on New Biology

Alphabetical List of Boxed Topics

Boxes provide supplemental content that is related to the topics in the chapters. These compartments help organize information so that "extras" can be scanned at a glance.

In alphabetical order, here are topics you'll find in boxes:

Notes

Part 1

Introduction

Notes

1

Accidental Cure

*Extreme medicine
for extreme patients.*

Have you ever wondered why some people who eat organic whole foods, exercise, have a positive mental attitude, and take nutritional supplements suffer from sudden heart attacks or from chronic, lingering illnesses? How about people who are diagnosed with cancer whom you thought were in good health? Doctors may run batteries of lab tests and come to the conclusion that a patient is physically fit, yet the patient may suffer from unexplainable debilitating fatigue, irritability, mood swings, or migrating pain.

Missing Link in Traditional Evaluations

If you're out of tune and out of balance but have perfect lab tests, there may be a missing link in your medical evaluation. Medical doctors may relieve symptoms with medications but they seldom offer solutions to correct the underlying problems. When a doctor is in doubt, he/she often blames genetics or calls the symptoms "idiopathic," meaning they don't know what is wrong. In desperation, a physician may even say a patient is malingering—meaning he/she is faking an illness to avoid work. At times, a doctor may also say an illness is "all in his/her head."

Treating the Symptoms of Disease

I have been practicing Internal Medicine for over 25 years, and I have been one of those physicians. I also worked for an HMO

(Health Management Organization) for almost 10 years before I recognized that I was treating the symptoms of disease with medications. The medications I prescribed have similar names that all begin with "anti" including antihypertensive, antiangina, antiinflammatory, antihypercholesterolemia or antiaging hormone replacements. The medications never correct the underlying problems and each medication creates its own side effects that require other medications. Such treatment creates a drug dependency and medications become medical intervention for the management of a disease. In an HMO, the management of a disease is lucrative business. Curing a patient is not financially rewarding for the medical-pharmaceutical industry.

Most of My Patients Have Embraced Natural Healing

As I started to investigate alternative, natural healing therapies, I began to write educational articles for my patients on preventive medicine. At the time I started writing, I was still working in a managed care practice, and most of my patients were very open and happy that their medical doctor was embracing natural healing methods. Now that I have been writing for over 15 years, I have decided to turn my articles into a book. This book is intended to uncover many underlying, hidden problems that most people do not know exist. The book will also challenge most readers' existing beliefs—especially with concepts from the field of energy medicine that includes biocybernetics and Acupuncture Meridian Assessment. Finally, the book will show how hidden dental problems, heavy metal toxicity, parasites, food allergies, and nutritional deficiency play an important role in so-called "incurable" medical problems.

An Opportunity for Accidental Cure Must Be Created

Two of my favorite articles are called "Accidental Cure" and "Extreme Medicine for Extreme Patients." I have decided to use the words "accidental healing" (that officially includes placebo effects and spontaneous healing) because such "accidents" are a lot more common than you may think. What's important to realize is that an opportunity for an "accidental cure" must be created in order for it to happen. In order to do this, one must first understand the biological "terrain" or condition of the body as a whole.

Our mind/body/spirit is unique and infinitely more complex than modern science can comprehend. When an "incurable" patient gets well by some form of healing other than what traditional medicine has to offer, doctors often attribute it to a placebo effect or a spontaneous healing. Sometimes, a medical professional will even go into denial by saying that they think they made a wrong diagnosis.

Acupuncture Meridian Assessment

Our bodies operate in several different energy realms including electrical and magnetic systems, as well as the familiar biomechanical and biochemical system. Although electrical and magnetic energies are used in diagnostic tools such as EKG (electrocardiogram) and MRI (magnetic resonance imaging), these tools operate using a "mechanistic" Newtonian view of the body. In addition to these diagnostic tools, there are other ways of measuring the "energy systems" of the body. I measure the energy in the body's acupuncture meridians—or the subtle human energies—in all my patients during their first visit. Acupuncture has been practiced for several thousand years in China and throughout Asia. Currently, the best science cannot explain the origin of the energy in the body's acupuncture meridians. Acupuncture Meridian Assessment, although not considered to be a diagnostic test, can reveal unique biofeedback information about a patient's energy patterns based on ancient knowledge of acupuncture and meridian flow of the body.

Imbalances in the Body's Biocybernetic System

When used by an experienced practitioner, the instrument used for Acupuncture Meridian Assessment detects electrical disturbance signals that can indicate hidden dental problems, environmental toxicities, hidden parasite infections, and other "imbalances" in the body. These "imbalances" are indications that the biocybernetic system is compromised and not functioning to its optimum capacity.

When you read the chapter on Acupuncture Meridian Assessment and "new" medicine based on ancient principles, it will give you a better understanding of the human body as a delicate energy system that might be considered analogous to a fine musical instrument such as a violin. The body, it may be said, is part of the symphony of Life.

Recommendations That May Seem Odd...

My assessment and recommendations may seem odd for some patients, and they may also provoke doubt and skepticism. For example, based on Acupuncture Meridian Assessment, a physical exam, laboratory tests, and a medical history, an extraction of an asymptomatic root canal may be recommended and a patient's arthritis or chest pain may improve. For another patient, a treatment for parasites may improve not only the patient's abdominal pain or irritable bowel but may also relieve the patient's knee pain, sciatic pain, or headache. In some people diagnosed with multiple sclerosis (MS), a treatment for parasites may even dissolve brain lesions.

Another patient may receive EDTA chelation therapy for heavy metal toxicity and their chest pain may go away. For yet another patient, when one or a combination of the above seemingly unrelated therapies are carried out, cancer may go into "spontaneous" remission. These phenomena are very difficult to explain by a deductionistic,

Newtonian-based western medical science. Our body/mind/spirit operates as a whole system, not simply a collection of parts. It operates in a closed biomechanical/chemical/electrical system within an open biocybernetic energy field.

Assessing the Whole System

On your first visit, I may not focus on your list of complaints or symptoms. You may think I am ignoring your complaints, but I am trying to create a "pattern" of the body's energy system based on Acupuncture Meridian Assessment. Rather than looking at your "collection of symptoms," I look at your entire system to correct any "disturbed" or "imbalanced" meridians. The body's immune system tries to heal itself as long as input and output are corrected.

Be warned: your medical problems may not be what you think or what you have been told. Discovering and correcting the underlying problems allows your body to heal itself regardless of your diagnosis. I call this healing phenomenon "accidental cure." Having experienced it first-hand, I know that this process works. The first time a patient witnesses this process, they are often surprised, amazed, and delighted. It is only then that they truly understand this phenomenon. If you can identify the underlying causes of your problems and balance the meridians, you may achieve an "accidental cure."

Medicine Among Ancient Societies

Every advanced society has had traditional medical care since the time of antiquity. The civilizations of Egypt, Greece, India, and China each had their own unique medical problems and distinct traditional medical practices. Today "standard medical care" of the ancients are referred to as Egyptian Antiquity Medicine, Greek Medicine, Ayurvedic Medicine, and Traditional Chinese Medicine.

Hippocrates is most known in western medicine for his Hippocratic Corpus and the Hippocratic Oath. Hippocratic physicians practiced medicine with limited medical knowledge. To them, healing was patient oriented with a focus on rebalancing the "dis-ease" of the patient, rather than overcoming the disease. For example, faced with a fever, one of the most dreaded medical conditions at the time, Hippocratic physicians did not attempt any heroic treatment. They gave general support with boiled barley water, honey, vinegar, and bedside attention.

Hippocratic Physicians Considered Drugs to be Unpredictable

Hippocratic physicians believed in the healing power of nature (Vis medicatrix naturae in Latin). Drug therapy was considered unpredictable, and these physicians preferred dietary regulation. A most notable quote from the Hippocratic philosophy reads:

> *Let your food be your medicine,*
> *let your medicine be your food.*

In his book, *Epidemics*, Hippocrates wrote:

> *... As to diseases, make*
> *a habit of two things—to help, or*
> *at least to do no harm.*

Hippocrates also realized that extreme remedies were sometimes necessary:

> *What drugs will not cure, the knife will;*
> *what the knife will not cure, the cautery will;*
> *what the cautery will not cure must be considered incurable.*

Some patients required potent medications to purge and expel excess black bile, and blood-letting was performed to establish balance in the body.

Patients Who Are Candidates for Extreme Medicine

Many patients come to see me with a whole list of medical conditions and unusual complaints. They have seen numerous medical doctors and alternative/complementary/holistic practitioners of different disciplines. Some of these patients come to see me with the self-claim, "Doctor, I am weird! Nobody knows what is wrong with me."

Doctors have often labeled these patients as difficult, extreme, or weird. Many of these patients are desperate to regain their life back. They're looking for "whatever it takes" to get well. These patients are good candidates for what I call, "extreme medicine for extreme patients" or "extraordinary medicine for extraordinary patients."

So, what is considered to be "extreme medicine" in today's standard medical care? Is it acupuncture or yoga? Not really. Some women will go through a preventive double mastectomy based on a family history of breast cancer and genetic testing. That is what I call extreme medicine. Heart bypass operations or heart transplants might have been considered extreme medicine 30 years ago, but by today's standards, these operations are considered no big deal. Chemotherapy, radiation therapy, and bone marrow transplants for cancer patients are also considered to be standard treatments by today's standards.

The definition of "extreme medicine" seems related to what a physician considers to be outside of his/her current *standard medical care*. For example, naturopathic medical doctors are mortified to see cancer patients go through chemo, radiation therapy, and bone marrow transplants. To them, it's as if a cancer patient is bombarded with napalm or nuked with a mini atomic bomb. For naturopathic physicians, today's accepted medical care is extreme medicine. I practice integrative extreme medicine every day for people who are considered to be extreme patients.

Standard Medical Treatment in My Office...

Although most physicians ridicule alternative medical doctors when they prescribe herbs to clean out the bowel, liver, and kidney, most of my patients start with bowel cleansing, kidney and liver cleansing, as well as parasite cleansing. Patients are also evaluated and mapped out for their cybernetic energy matrix based on an Acupuncture Meridian Assessment. Hair tissue mineral analysis and food allergy tests are also standards that are used to design nutritional and dietary recommendations.

For more complex extreme patients, biological terrain assessment (BTA), computerized regulation thermography (CRT) or infrared thermography, Heidelberg pH gastric analysis, dark field microscopy blood analysis, electro interstitial scan (EIS), and heart rate variability (HRV) tests are performed to sort out the underlying biological disturbances. Often, IV (intravenous) chelation therapy, IV nutritional therapy, hyperbaric oxygen therapy, ozone therapy, or bio-resonance therapy are added. Gallbladder/liver flush are also required for all my difficult, extreme, or weird patients.

Spontaneous Healing or Accidental Cure

When you apply all these unusual modalities and therapies in the right sequence, you'll often observe spontaneous healing or an accidental cure. The body begins to repair and correct itself when you remove underlying toxic conditions, such as heavy metals, hidden infections, and allergies.

Having an unexplained medical condition does not mean you're weird. However, you might be a candidate for the extreme medicine that I have described, or extraordinary medicine for extraordinary patients. You'll also need a physician who is knowledgeable about many unusual alternative therapies. Hopefully, he isn't too weird.

I hope this chapter excites you and prepares you to explore new concepts: biological terrain, Acupuncture Meridian Assessment, biocybernetics, chelation therapy for heavy metal toxicity, dental-medical connections, parasites, food allergies, nutritional therapy, detoxification, and much more. After you read the book's first three chapters, then jump to a special interest topic and uncover your own journey toward an *Accidental Cure*.

Patient Testimonial and Success Story
Kidney Cancer Follow-up:
Building the Immune System

Since starting with Dr. Yu, we discovered I had mercury toxicity, parasites, and weakened organ functions. In my alternative medicine research, I found that these are a few of the many causes of a weakened immune system that can lead to cancer or a variety of other illnesses. These "weak links" of my body have been remedied through the following actions: replacement of all my mercury fillings, chelation for the removal of mercury in my body, parasite cleansing, and nutritional support to strengthen weak organ function as well as build my immune system.

For more of this patient's case history and testimonial, see page 289.

Notes

2

Biological Terrain and Biocybernetic Medicine

The concept of the biological terrain compares the body to a mini-ecosystem that is influenced by several biological factors.

Biocybernetic medicine identifies light (photons) as a vehicle that carries biological information that encourages cells to heal.

This chapter groups together two concepts that are cornerstones of my practice. Because of medical politics, the concept of biological terrain is foreign to conventionally trained medical doctors, and biocybernetic medicine is a cutting-edge concept that has become popular with alternative medical doctors in Europe. Hence, both concepts are little known among conventionally trained medical doctors in the United States.

The Health of the Body's Internal Environment

The concept for biological terrain has been around for many years. It originated with a contemporary of Louis Pasteur's named Claude Bernard (1813-1878) who developed the idea that the body's ability to heal is dependent on its internal environment. Although Bernard developed the original concept of the biological terrain, a medical doctor named Antoine Béchamp (1816-1908) is largely responsible for a more complete theory of biological terrain. Béchamp built on Bernard's idea and said that health and disease revolve around a concept called "pleomorphism." While Pasteur was promoting the idea that disease is due to single, fixed-state microbes, Béchamp discovered tiny microorganisms that are "pleomorphic" or "many formed." Pleomorphic microorganisms are found to be present in all things, whether living or dead. In Béchamp's view, these microorganisms are capable of taking on a number of forms, and the forms depend on the chemistry of their environment (the body of the host), or the biological terrain.

Modern Medicine Favored Pasteur—Due to Antimicrobials

Pasteur is most known for his germ theory that became the foundation of modern medicine, mostly due to the wide use of antimicrobial remedies. In the second half of the nineteeth century, Louis Pasteur, a French chemist, competed with a German doctor named Robert Koch in an odd "Franco-German" microbial war in which the scientists worked diligently to prove that their respective country was superior. In 1885, Pasteur's goal was to solve the problem of human disease, and he developed a successful vaccine for rabies. As a result of this achievement, newspapers funded the Pasteur Institute in Paris that made Pasteur the victor. Indirectly, the rivalry between Pasteur and Koch produced a method for making vaccines and solidified the theory that microbes caused disease.

Understanding Biological Terrain

Today, many scientists understand that Pasteur's germ theory is misguided. In contrast to Pasteur, Bernard and Béchamp believed that disease is a function of biology, and illness is the result of multiple changes that take place in the body when metabolic processes are thrown off. Germs are actually symptoms of a weakened terrain that becomes vulnerable to harmful microorganisms.

A biological terrain may be compared to a garden that requires an understanding of soil conditions. Gardeners who grow healthy fruits and vegetables understand that a plant's environment will determine whether the plant is healthy. They know that a garden is much more than a plot of land where seeds are planted. A healthy crop also requires an in-depth knowledge of the seeds, nutrients, fertilizers, water drainage, and sunlight. It also requires an understanding of how insects, weeds, molds, and fungi affect the soil and plants.

Managing a healthy biological terrain in the human body is similar to raising healthy vegetables. If the body is fed a diet that provides adequate amounts of vitamins and minerals, if it is nurtured with love and given an adequate amount of exercise, rest, and sleep, the body, like a healthy garden, can flourish with vitality and support a strong immune system. When your immune system is strong and your biological terrain is balanced, you can ward off infections and stay healthy.

The Use of Antibiotics Has Led to the Development of Super Bugs

Pasteur's germ theory is the foundation of modern medicine's triumph over infectious diseases, but it is also the cause of antibiotic resistance and the development of new and emerging super bugs. The germ theory states that germs are airborne, and specific germs cause specific diseases. This theory led to treatment plans that are designed to eliminate what is believed to be the underlying problem —the disease-causing germs.

Holistic Medicine Sees the Biological Terrain as the Cause of Disease

Medicine's reaction to a patient with *Streptococcus bacillus* provides an example of the difference between the conventional medical approach that is based on the germ theory and a holistic approach that focuses on the biological terrain. *Streptococcus bacillus* is believed to be the cause of an infectious strep throat, which is indicated by a positive throat culture, as well as the symptoms of sore throat, swollen lymph nodes, and a fever. The most common treatment includes the use of an antibiotic to kill off as many strep-tococci as possible. Typically, aspirin or Tylenol is also prescribed to control the fever and painful sore throat. When the patient's fever and sore throat subside within a few days, the doctor and patient are both happy about the quick response to medications.

In contrast to Pasteur's theory, holistic medicine sees the environment of the body or the biological terrain as the cause of disease. In the holistic view, *Streptococcus bacillus* is not the cause of the strep throat. Instead, a breakdown in the immune system creates an environment for the *Streptococcus* to transform into an infectious, virulent form. The breakdown of the immune system is caused by a disturbance of the biological terrain and the factors that trigger the disrupted biological terrain may not be familiar to you or your doctor (See: Stressors That Can Disturb Your Biological Terrain).

Professor Vincent's Biological Terrain Score

In the 1920s, a French researcher named Professor Vincent developed specific electrical parameters that correlate with the conditions of the biological terrain. The following parameters (assessed from the blood, saliva, and urine) yield what Vincent considered to be a "biological terrain score" that can be used to predict an individual's susceptibility to general illness, fatigue, or degenerative conditions:

- Value of pH (acidity or alkalinity)

- Oxidation-reduction potential (electron movement or free radical activity)

- Resistivity (opposition to the passage of a steady electrical current)

Through Corrective Action—The Body Will Heal Itself

From a holistic point of view, the *Streptococcus* described in our example, has an important role to play in the restoration of the biological terrain. This bug produces a fever, mucous, and a cough as a means to activate the innate natural immune response and activate a built-in cleansing program. In a sense, the *Streptococcus* is not your enemy but a facilitator that accomplishes a natural balance in the body. This perspective emphasizes a need to correct the underlying conditions that weaken the immune system by providing:

- Proper rest and sleep
- Stress control
- Nutritional support with extra vitamins, minerals, and herbs
- Proper oral/dental care (a primary source of *Streptococcus*) if indicated.

Through these corrective actions, the body will heal itself by restoring its proper biological terrain. With enough support, the body will overcome the hardship of the *Streptococcus* fever, inflammation, and pain.

Antibiotics Will Only Prolong the Disease Process

The idea that *Streptococcus* is a messenger that gives your body an early warning to take corrective actions is unfamiliar to most people and their doctors. Using antibiotics and suppressing the fever will only prolong the disease process by interfering with the body's ability to heal itself. Antibiotics and aspirin (or Tylenol) are rarely indicated in the holistic view due to the fact that they can suppress the body's natural immune response.

Germs are not the cause of the disease, but appear only after a person has become ill. They are created by nature to assist in eliminating our toxins and waste. The difference between treating the symptoms with allopathic medications to counter and mask the symptoms versus treating the underlying causes has profound implications—especially for treating chronic disease. Chronic diseases such as cancer, heart disease, strokes, diabetes, and new emerging medical conditions do not fit into the classical model of modern science, and patients are beginning to understand that conventional medicine is not equipped to treat these degenerative diseases. More and more, my patients tell me, "If my doctor said everything is fine, why do I feel so bad?" To understand why we get sick, we need to understand the "terrain."

What Is pH?

pH is a measure of the acidity or alkalinity of a solution, and a roll of pH paper provides a means to monitor the health of your terrain (See: "Monitoring the Health of Your Biological Terrain"). The acronym pH is an abbreviation for "potential hydrogen," which refers to the concentration of hydrogen ions:

- **Acidic pH**
  Low, or acidic pH values are solutions with high concentrations of hydrogen ions (H+). Acids have a pH less than 7 (or more hydrogen ions than water).

- **Alkaline pH**
  High pH values are solutions called "bases" that have low concentrations of hydrogen ions. Bases have a pH greater than 7 (or less hydrogen ions than water).

Environmental pollution, food processing, and the toxic chemicals found in food, are just a few of the factors that have an acidic effect on the body (See: "Stressors That Can Disturb Your Biological Terrain").

Micro Essentials Laboratory has been selling pH papers for several decades. Single rolls are available online or at health food stores (See: "Source for Buying pH Paper").

Source for Buying pH Paper

pH Paper, Single-Roll Dispenser (#067)
pH 5.5 - 8.0

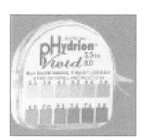

Micro Essential Laboratory
Brooklyn, New York 11210
(718) 338-3618
www.microessentiallab.com

Biocybernetics Is a Hot Topic in Europe

Biocybernetics is an up-and-coming hot topic in the new emerging field of European energy medicine. Biocybernetic medicine is actually not a new idea but an old concept that has been given a new name. A biocybernetic matrix is a modern term for the meridian system in acupuncture and the related field of Acupunture Meridian Assessment developed by Reinhold Voll, M.D., in Germany in the 1950s.

In November 2006, I attended the International Symposium of Biocybernetic Medicine in Germany. The symposium included medical doctors, acupuncturists, and natural medical doctors as well as engineers, physicists, and mathematicians who developed an instrument that detect how cells communicate with each other.

Professor Fritz-Albert Popp, Ph.D.

Professor Fritz-Albert Popp, Ph.D., a theoretical physicist and biophysicist from Germany, is considered to be the father of the bio-photon theory. A biophoton is a photon of light that is emitted from a biological system that can be detected with biological probes.

Stressors That Can Disturb Your Biological Terrain

The most common stressors that can disturb your biological terrain are:

- **Poor Diet and Nutrition**
  The average American consumes over 150 pounds of sugar, mainly in a form of high fructose corn syrup that has been associated with an epidemic rise in obesity and diabetes. Too many processed, chemical-laden, convenience foods can destroy your biological terrain and your health.

- **Lack of Adequate High-Quality Water**
  In the 1950s, the French government found a region with an alarming rate of cancer, and they commissioned Professor Vincent to find the cause. He determined that the water was the main culprit. The water in the region had been oxidized. It was acidic and blocked metabolic detoxification. The most cost-effective way to purify water is to use a charcoal-based filtration system that filters tap water.

- **Psychological Stress and Negative Emotions**
  Over ten billion doses of tranquilizers, antidepressants, barbiturates, and amphetamines are prescribed each year. There are also an estimated 50,000 stress-related suicides each year (only one in eight attempts are successful). Stress has a direct negative effect on your psycho-neuro-endocrine and immune systems.

- **Medical Therapy and Medications**
  Over 225,000 deaths have been identified as iatrogenic (medical therapy related). As of the year 2000, this has become the third leading cause of death, after heart disease and cancer. (Starfield B. Is U.S. health really the best in the world? *JAMA*. 2000; 284(4):483-485.)

- **Environmental Poisoning and Heavy Metal Toxicity**
  To understand environmental pollution, it is helpful to read the eye-opening issue on environmental pollution in a *National Geographic* cover story titled "Chemicals Within Us," published in the October 2006 issue.
  An online version is available on the *National Geographic* Web site at: http://science.nationalgeographic.com/science/health-and-human-body/human-body/chemicals-within-us.html.

- **Hidden Dental Problems**
  The magnitude of dental-related medical problems is huge, yet this is ignored by both the medical and dental professions because dental and medical problems are viewed as separate and unrelated. In reality, they are complex dental/medical or medical/dental problems. Examples include:

  - Root canals
  - Amalgams
  - Allergic reaction to dental materials
  - Galvanic currents in the mouth
  - Temporomandibular joint (TMJ) Note: The temporomandibular joint connects the lower jaw to the skull.
  - Bite problems
  - Periodontal infections
  - Cavitation—an infection in the jaw bone

  Hidden dental problems have became a "no man's land" due to the fact that they are not addressed by medical doctors or dentists. At the same time, they have become critical obstacles to getting well and to correcting a biological terrain. In my experience, it is only through the collaboration of an experienced medical doctor and a dentist that a patient has a chance to fix his/her hidden dental and related medical problems. Both the doctor and the dentist need to understand the meridian systems and use biocybernetic technology.

- **Parasites and New Emerging Infections**
  Global warming and the global migration of human beings have changed the whole perspective of geographically isolated disease. Most people associate parasites with the third world (or the politically correct global south), but the problem is now pervasive worldwide.

- **Allergies**
  The incidence of allergies is rapidly rising in developed countries, and the underlying problems are an implication of the broad spectrum of changes in the environmental terrain. Allergy is a misdirected, inappropriate immune response, and one of the most neglected areas is an unsuspected delayed immune response (IgG reaction) to food allergies from the food we eat every day.

- **Inactivity**
  Balance of *motion* and *emotion* is related to the balance of life.

- **Vaccinations**
  Too many vaccinations are given to young infants at too early an age. Although the politics of vaccinations is beyond the scope of this book, it suffices to say that vaccinations have been associated with autism and auto-immune diseases.

- **Structural Imbalance**
  Structural imbalance of the body refers to the body's skeletal system that can be aggravated by stress or malnutrition.

- **Lack of Natural Sunlight and Cosmic Rays**
  Inactivity and life indoors leads to a deficiency in natural sunlight and cosmic rays—especially in winter months.

- **Electromagnetic Pollution**
  Electromagnetic pollution interferes with the biocybernetic field of living organisms from bees to mankind. It manifests as new and emerging medical problems, especially in young children who are highly susceptible to electromagnetic pollution.

- **Genetically Modified Organisms (GMOs)**
  The consumption of genetically modified food is an unknown danger for future generations. You are what you eat: genetically modified food will create a genetically modified human. I highly recommend Jeffrey M. Smith's *Seeds of Deception* that exposes the dark secrets of GMOs.

- **Scars**
  Major surgical scars or minor childhood scars, such as tonsillectomy or scars from an accident, may block the energy flow of the main meridians and create unusual medical symptoms.

Popp's work on biophotons actually goes back to Russia in the 1920s when Russian embryologist Alexander Gurwitsch reported "ultra-weak" photon emissions from living tissues in the ultraviolet range of the spectrum. Fritz Popp and a young graduate student named Bernard Ruth took Gurwitsch's work much further when they built a high-sensitivity emission photometer that was capable of mapping the light or biophotons given off by living systems. They counted biophotons given off by test substances and discovered:

- Vegetables contaminated with heavy metals showed a decreased photon count.

- Tomatoes stored at cold temperatures showed decreased biophoton emissions that decreased even further with longer storage times.

- Photons given off by eggs from captive chickens was lower than from eggs obtained from free-range chickens.

Popp also measured biophotons given off from the human body and saw high photon emissions coming from the hands of an internationally acclaimed healer named Rosalyn Bruyere when she focused her healing energy compared to light given off when she was resting. Popp suspected that the source of these biophotons was DNA and theorized that each organ and each cell has its own specific spectra, as well as specific disease-producing oscillations with characteristic frequencies. Note: Oscillation refers to a cycle associated with the wave phenomena of light.

Monitoring the pH of Your Biological Terrain

In a healthy person, a saliva pH reading should be 6.5 - 6.75 most of the time. People with either chronic degenerative diseases or those on the way to degenerative disease will see wake-up saliva from 5.5 or lower with urine pH as low as 4.5. Low pH values reflect a long-term acid stress on the body representing low alkaline reserves that are very low to depleted.

When you eat a meal, the saliva pH should rise to 7.2.
A low pH reading during a meal is also a reflection of low alkaline reserves.

Urine pH Reading After an Acid-Forming Meal

Meat, pasta, beans, bread, nuts, and fish are all acid-forming. If you check your morning urine pH after an acid-forming meal:

- **pH Reading of 4.5 to 5.8**
  This range reflects adrenals and kidneys that have enough energy to buffer and dispose of the acid from the meal.

- **pH reading of 6.8 or Higher**
  If your morning pH after an acid-forming meal is 6.8 or higher, it is possible that the body is dumping bicarbonate ions in the ammonia cycle of the liver to help deal with the acid. This situation may mean depleted alkaline reserves, possible exhausted adrenal glands, and digestive problems.

Saliva pH Reading After an Acid-Forming Meal

If your morning urine pH is off and your morning saliva pH is less than 5.8, your alkaline reserve levels are critically low. The further apart the pH numbers are, the more sick you are.

Urine pH Reading After an Alkaline-Forming Meal

After an evening meal of mostly vegetables, if you check your morning urine pH:

- **pH Reading of 4.5 to 5.5**
  This range is too acid after an alkaline-forming meal reflecting a lot of stored acidity. More alkaline-forming foods are advised.

- **pH Reading of 5.5 to 6.8**
  This range could be fine if you feel healthy. If you have health problems, it could mean that your alkaline reserves are being dumped due to an underlying imbalance or toxicity problem.

The preservation of the healthy oscillation is dependent on the resonating capacity of the cell, organ, tissue, or the whole body, and when the resonating capacity is disturbed, incoherent, inappropriate, disease can develop. Popp discovered that disease has its own electromagnetic waves and traced tumor problems back to a loss of coherence in the biophoton field.

All Living Organisms Possess Complex Electromagnetic Fields

The new breakthrough in medicine will come from understanding the biophysics and biocybernetics of cells and organs, not from the *Human Genome Project*. Here's what scientists know about the biocybernetics of cells and organs:

- All living organisms possess complex electromagnetic fields and an invisible body

- Biophotons trigger all biochemical reactions in the living cell

- Electromagnetic fields disappear completely with death

Electromagnetic Oscillations

Dr. Franz Morell, M.D., from Germany (who died in 1990) said, "The oscillation (frequency) of the universe is the cause of the phenomenon called LIFE. These oscillations bring both health and disease. Without electromagnetic oscillations, life is probably inconceivable. Oscillations have four dimensions: length, width, height, and time. Self-healing requires an active cancellation of pathological oscillations and a rebalancing of a disturbed equilibrium. Here are some interesting points that connect the oscillations in biocybernetics with acupuncture meridians:

- An information exchange within a living organism can only be transmitted by oscillations that move at the speed of light (Popp).

- We are living in the matrix of a biocybernetic system.

- The oscillations of the organs are present on the acupuncture points in a bunched and concentrated form.

- The frequency spectrum of an organ is conducted via the meridians and can be detected at the acupuncture points. Nearly the whole oscillation spectrum of the body exists in the palms of the hands or the soles of the feet.

Invisible Body Map of the Biocybernetic Matrix

To my amazement, we already have "an invisible body map of the biocybernetic matrix" in the acupuncture meridian system taught in traditional Chinese medicine (TCM) and the chakra system taught in Ayurvedic medicine. Acupuncture Meridian Assessment (AMA), also known as electroacupuncture according to Dr. Voll (EAV), is one of the most effective ways to learn about the biocybernetic system because it provides a physical means to measure invisible energy functions unknown to Western medicine.

When you can measure the biological terrain and understand the biocybernetic regulation of the body, you can detect hidden dental infections, parasites, allergies, and toxins building up in your body and start a treatment plan that seems almost impossible in the context of current medical science. All of this makes my type of practice seem magical for some new patients and highly suspicious to my medical colleagues in academia or clinical practice. For me, the biocybernetic medicine component of my practice is fascinating, fun, and rewarding. Best of all, it never gets boring.

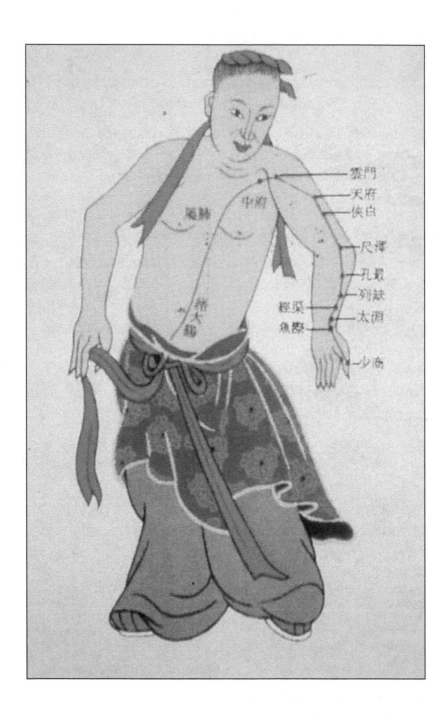

Patient Testimonial
Multiple Symptoms Other Doctors' Tests
Could Not Diagnose

My immune system really took a dip and I developed mono-nucleosis. I was sent to numerous doctors, mostly diagnosing me with asthma, chronic fatigue, and sinusitis directly from the mold. Scariest of all—I was diagnosed with demyelination of the central nervous system due to what the doctors think to be a prolonged suppressed immune system.

(...)

Dr. Yu treated me for several issues to improve. My husband, family, friends and co-workers were amazed at how I was recovering.

For more of this patient's case history and testimonial, see page 307.

Notes

3

Acupuncture Meridian Assessment (AMA)

*Curing the incurable by measuring
the immeasurable.*

In my practice, I explain to new patients that I compare a
human body that is sick to a violin that is out of tune. This makes
a doctor the person who does the tuning. The medical name
I give to the job of tuning is Acupuncture Meridian Assessment
(AMA). As you'll discover in this chapter, a violin metaphor helps
explain the concept of energy medicine that is not widely understood
in the United States.

For the purpose of explaining AMA, the violin has the following
characteristics that make it analogous to the human body:

- **Four Strings**
  The four strings on a violin have a conceptual resemblance to
  the human body's 50 major acupuncture meridians.

- **Components That Produce Sound**
  The EAV device that is used for Acupuncture Meridian Assessment and the strings on a violin both produce sound. The vibrations of the strings on the violin are transferred to the body of the
  violin, and the sound radiates into the air. The subtle vibrational
  energy measured at acupoints on the body is also transferred to the
  EAV device that produces sounds. It is really not the strings or the

acupoints themselves that produce sound, but the interaction with other components (the body of the violin and the EAV device).

- **Need for Tuning or Pitch Adjustment**
  The violin and the body both have a need for tuning (See: "What is Tuning or Pitch Adjustment?"). Although tuning on the human body may some day be accomplished with techniques that are as easy as turning the pegs on a violin, today tuning is accomplished with:

  1. *A Meridian Assessment*
     A meridian assessment is accomplished with a Voll machine or electroacupuncture according to Voll (EAV) device. This diagnostic tool measures the flow of energy to organs via acupoint voltages measured on the hands and feet.

  2. *Alternative or Conventional Medical Treatment*
     The EAV device provides a clue that helps me treat a patient with an alternative or conventional medical therapy, depending on the severity of the illness.

  3. *One or More Follow-up Meridian Assessments*
     As the body heals, the voltages measured at acupuncture points move toward normal *baseline* electrical voltages developed by Dr. Reinhard Voll.

- **Complex Anatomy**
  The violin and the body have a complex internal and external anatomy made of natural materials that are sensitive to the environment.

- **Proper Care Is Required Due to Perpetual Vibration**
  With use, the body and the violin both experience physical changes that are due to vibration. Although vibrational energy is a relatively new concept in the field of Western medicine, the body is really composed of energy that vibrates at different frequencies or rates of vibration. With proper care, the body and the violin can facilitate a life-long journey of gratifying experiences.

Acupuncture Meridian Assessment Does Not Use Needles

It is quite common for new patients to assume that there are needles involved in the Acupuncture Meridian Assessment work that I do. My work with the EAV device measures skin resistivity at 54 of the 500 classical acupuncture points, and there are no needles involved. Organs and teeth are all connected to the acupuncture meridians. Physical symptoms in the body are reflected in the mouth, and biological dentists understand the connection between weak organs and problem teeth. The points that I measure run along the system of channels or major meridians that feed energy to the organs of the body.

A *New York Times* Reporter Introduced Acupuncture to the West

Although traditional acupuncture is thought to have originated in China several thousand years ago, Americans did not become aware of acupuncture until 1971. In that year, James Reston, a *New York Times* reporter, described a doctor's use of acupuncture to help relieve his postoperative pain after an emergency appendectomy in China. During

---

Famous Violin Maker Families

The first true ancestor of the 4-string violin was made in northern Italy in 1550 by Giovan Giacomo della Corna that was later perfected by the Amati family of Cremona.

Antonia Stradivarius, who is believed to have studied in the Amati workshops, is thought to have produced some of the finest violins ever made. Andrea Guarneri, who was an apprentice in the workshop of Nicolo Amati, also produced violins whose quality is considered comparable to those of the Amati and Stradivari families.

What Is Tuning or Pitch Adjustment?

Unless you play a string instrument, you may not be familiar with tuning. String instruments, such as the violin and guitar, need tuning to adjust their strings to proper pitches.

Pitch (or frequency) refers to the number of vibrations per second of each note in the musical scale. The A string is usually a reference pitch that is tuned first. In 1939, the violin's A string (above Middle C) was defined as 440 vibrations per second as a standard, although some orchestras tune to another standard A, such as 442, or even as high as 445 or 446 Hz to produce a brighter sound.

Musicians tune their instruments by tightening or loosening each string. On a violin, this is accomplished by turning the pegs at the top of the violin or metal screws called fine tuners that fit into a flared piece of wood called the tailpiece. The tighter the string, the higher the pitch. Unlike pianos that can be tuned once or twice a year, violins (and guitars) need to be tuned before they are played. Temperature, humidity, and the type of music played can affect the strings, making it necessary to re-tune.

Richard Nixon's administration, while on a trip with Henry Kissinger, Chinese doctors removed Reston's inflamed appendix. When Reston experienced pain during the second night after his surgery, the Peking hospital's doctor of acupuncture inserted three thin needles into the outer part of his right elbow and below his knees. To stimulate the needles into action, the doctor lit two pieces of an herb and held them close to Reston's abdomen, while he occasionally twirled the needles. Reston reported that after 20 minutes, there was a

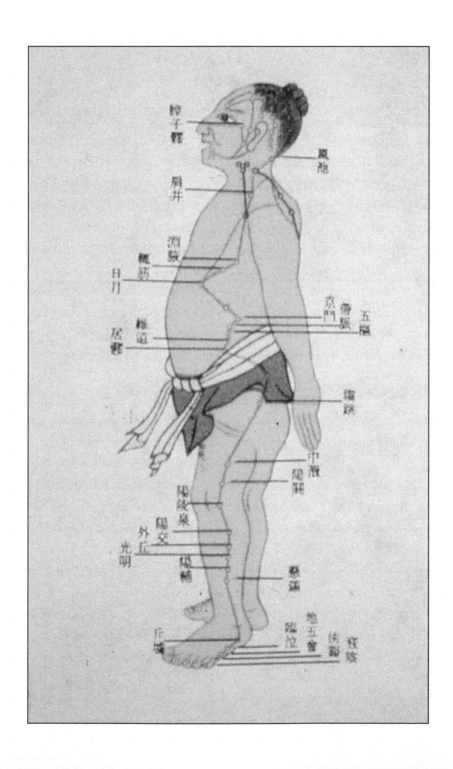

noticeable relaxation of the pressure and the distension in his abdomen had disappeared.

Acupuncture Has Never "Fit" into the Western Medical Model

Many doctors who heard about James Reston's experience with acupuncture in the 1970s dismissed it as a "placebo" effect that has been accepted by Western medicine since the beginning of the 20th century. Placebos are sugar pills or saline injections that are given to patients in place of drugs and result in therapeutic improvement. The improvement is thought to be due to a patient's faith in their doctor. Because Western doctors expect to see as many as 30 percent of patients have therapeutic improvement with a "pharmacologically inert substance," they were quick to assume that acupuncture's benefits were due to placebo. The placebo effect does not explain acupuncture's success on animals, but this point is rarely discussed in the West.

Technological Verification of the Existence of Meridians

Western medicine has tried to explain acupuncture in the context of an established human physiology model that includes the nerves of the body, hormones, and the body's biochemistry. Soviet scientists in the 1970s were the first to study electrical characteristics of acupuncture points. Although European and American doctors were never able to identify anatomical components of a meridian, a Korean doctor named Dr. Kim Bong Han identified meridian pathways using radioactive tracers in rabbits in the 1960s. Dr. Kim's work was later confirmed by Drs. Claude Darra and Pierre De Vernejoul in an experiment using human subjects in the early 1980s. While these experiments did not prove the existence of a life energy that the Chinese refer to as ch'i (pronounced chee), a technological verification of the existence of meridians has helped lay the groundwork for the acceptance of energy medicine in the medical community.

Curing the Incurable by Measuring the Immeasurable: Mapping the Invisible Body by Biocybernetics

Although I've placed most of my published articles in Part 3, this article, published in *The Healthy Planet* magazine, fits very well into this chapter.

≈ ≈ ≈

Is it possible to map the invisible body? In Germany, there is an emerging biomedical discipline called biocybernetics, which has been measuring the invisible energy field of the human body. Biocybernetics is a key component of the broader field of energy medicine in Europe. It is actually not a new idea but an old concept that has been given a new name. A biocybernetic matrix is a modern term for the acupuncture meridian system and the related field of Acupuncture Meridian Assessment developed by Reinhold Voll, M.D., in the 1950s in Germany.

In 1895, German physicist Wilhelm C. Roentgen discovered mysterious rays capable of passing through the human body. Because of their unknown nature, he called them x-rays. Because of his discovery, he was awarded the first Nobel Prize in Physics in 1901. X-rays are electromagnetic waves situated between UV (ultraviolet) light and gamma rays on the wavelength scale. Marie Curie built x-ray machines for French doctors in World War I. It helped detect the location of bullets, shrapnel, and broken bones in the body, which, of course, were invisible to the human eye. X-rays revolutionized medicine, and the rest "became history." Measuring the "immeasurable" human energy field by utilizing the biocybernetic matrix of the body's meridian systems will have a similar impact.

Every day, I see patients who have been to one doctor after another, and one hospital after another, trying to figure out why they are so sick. None of the various specialists these patients have seen seem to have any clue as to what is wrong with them.

Marie, a 19-year-old college student, is an example. Her complaint was a history of chest and leg pain for over a year. Although she saw several cardiologists, an orthopedic surgeon, and other specialists, none of her doctors gave her a definite diagnosis or treatment plan, even after extensive medical tests and evaluations.

When I saw her, her physical exam was normal. I checked 54 acupuncture points as part of my meridian assessment evaluation. Out of the 54 points that I evaluated, her dental area meridian showed pathology. A further detailed evaluation revealed that her problem was arising from tooth number 17—an old wisdom tooth socket area.

Marie's problem was a dental-related medical problem, which is an all-too-common and all-too-often overlooked situation. Medical doctors cannot understand or fix her problem. She needs an oral surgeon to correct the problem. I could not guarantee that oral surgery would fix her chest and leg pain. However, based on over 15 years of practicing Acupuncture Meridian Assessments, I told her I was 85-90% confident that her symptoms would resolve when her dental problem was properly fixed.

This is not an isolated event. I've had multiple cases of unexplainable chest pain that respond favorably to cleaning out an old infected wisdom tooth area.

The power of biocybernetics and meridian assessment evaluations are used to reveal the true cause of underlying illnesses.

Once the true cause is revealed, a specific treatment plan can be implemented and, sometimes almost unbelievably, self-healing is achieved.

An elderly woman with fibromyalgia is another example. An evaluation revealed that her diagnosis of fibromyalgia wasn't really fibromyalgia. Her evaluation indicated that she should be treated with parasite medications. She fully responded and her unexplainable pain disappeared.

Another woman's asthma disappeared after an extraction of a root canal. Still another woman's asthma was eliminated with parasite medications. These two different women with the same condition (asthma) required two distinct approaches because the individual condition of each person was unique.

 A young woman with acute panic attacks and a nervous breakdown responded to the removal of her "silver" fillings and recovered her normal mental health. Note: Silver fillings are approximately 50% mercury.

None of these patients responded to traditional medical care because their medical evaluations weren't addressing the true cause of their ill health. Instead, they were simply heavily medicated to control their symptoms. They were considered incurable and advised to learn to live with their illness because doctors could not determine what was wrong with them.

Quite a few of my patients come from all over the United States. This includes a sizable group from Iowa who drive 7-8 hours to see me. They do so because they realize they are not getting better, even after going to the Mayo Clinic. After extensive visits to this Midwestern institution, they need a different outlook on their health and healing. I am always grateful to the Mayo Clinic for their extensive medical evaluations. They have one of the best medical systems available based on Western medical science, and they utilize every known test at their disposal.

After these individuals have been evaluated by the Mayo Clinic without a clear diagnosis, I have the opportunity to evaluate them from my "outside-of-the-box" viewpoint. I have repeatedly noticed an emerging pattern of overlooked causes in modern medical diagnosis. The most common neglected areas are hidden dental-related medical problems, heavy metal toxicity, nutritional deficiencies, parasite problems, and a general lack of understanding of the importance of detoxification of the colon, liver, and kidney.

How do I know these problems are the missing links? By understanding Biocybernetics and measuring the acupuncture meridian systems in the body's invisible energy matrix. The human body is like a fine-tuned musical instrument that requires constant tuning and calibration to keep one in optimal health.

We desperately need "connections for optimal health" or links that integrate Western-based medical science and the emerging knowledge of biocybernetics through Acupuncture Meridian Assessment. X-rays eventually became less mysterious and later contributed to major advancements in medicine. By combining these disciplines, we can truly "cure the incurable" by "measuring the immeasurable" human energy fields. Just as violins need to be tuned before they are played, the body needs similar tuning. Temperature, humidity, and the type of music played can also affect the strings, making it necessary to re-tune.

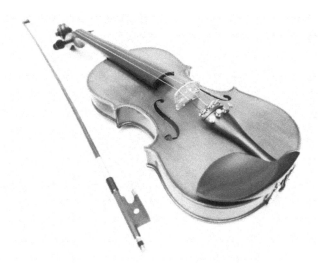

Patient Testimonial
Three Years of Bronchial Symptoms Resolved
in Three Months

I have been a relatively healthy person until about 3 years ago when I came down with recurring bronchitis and pneumonia from which I was unable to fully recover. Soon after, I was diagnosed with bronchiectasis, a condition where the lungs don't work properly to rid mucus from the airways.

(...)

It's been nearly 5 months since I first visited Dr. Yu, and I can tell you that I haven't felt this good in over 3 years. During my last two appointments, the Acupuncture Meridian Assessment indicated that all my meridians are in the normal range.

For more of this patient's case history and testimonial, see page 302.

Part 2

Staying Healthy in a Toxic World

Notes

4

Heavy Metals

Heavy metals mean heavy feelings:
Chelation therapy for toxic tuna and planet Earth

Tuna fish has been an inexpensive, tasty fish that Americans have loved for many years. Today, however, the Food and Drug Administration (FDA) and the Environmental Protection Agency (EPA) tell pregnant women to limit their tuna fish servings to six ounces per week. This is because of the possible mercury levels in tuna that can affect the neurological development of a fetus and young children.

Dead-End Responses From Doctors Concerning Mercury

If you are tired, depressed, and concerned about the possible effect of mercury on your nervous system and ask your doctor for a mercury level test due to your exposure to tuna fish, your doctor will probably dismiss the issue and write a prescription for an antidepressant medication. You will most likely get the same dead-end response for a similar concern about the mercury in your dental amalgams.

If you persist and convince your medical doctor to check your mercury level, he will order a blood test that will be negative, and his/her response will be "I told you so." The reason every blood test for mercury will be negative is because heavy metals, such as mercury, lead, and cadmium, accumulate in the organs and tissues—and not in the blood.

Metal Accumulates Over a Person's Lifetime

In the general population and in young children, lead toxicity is a lot more common than you may think. Whether you like it or not, we will accumulate many toxins during our lifetime — especially heavy metals. Sources include the environment, our diet, and often routine dental and medical care from amalgams and vaccinations. The consequences of this accumulation are the most severe in children due to their small body weight. Tests show that children are highly susceptible to neurologic developmental problems. Even at the lowest measurable lead level, lead toxicity demonstrates a reduced IQ in children. Research shows there is no safe level of lead (Richard L. Canfield, Ph.D. *New England Journal of Medicine*; 2002).

Heavy Metals Make You Feel Toxic

If you feel down, tired, anxious, or depressed, and all your standard medical tests are negative, heavy metal exposure might be the problem. The medical conditions associated with heavy metals are too vast to mention. Whether you are young or old, heavy metals have a direct toxic effect and will:

- Create oxidative stress and an inflammatory response that affect your psycho-neuro-immuno-endocrine system

- Contribute to medical conditions from autism in children to cancer and Alzheimer's in adults.

It is not uncommon to be exposed to several toxic metals, such as lead, mercury, tin, arsenic, nickel, aluminum, and cadmium. The magnitude of heavy-metal exposure has been downplayed by our medical community. We are not training our young physicians about "low-level" chronic heavy metal exposure and the biologic effects of heavy-metal toxicology. We are only teaching them how to treat symptoms with medications.

Hair Mineral Analysis and a Confirmation Chelation Challenge Test

I have discovered that the most cost-effective screening test for heavy metals is a hair tissue mineral analysis performed by a reputable lab. Mercury usually does not come out of your hair, especially mercury from dental amalgams and a hair mineral analysis is an indirect way to measure the accumulation in your organs and tissues. A hair tissue mineral analysis can be confirmed with a chelation challenge test that is accomplished with chelating agents. Chelating agents like dimercaptopropane sulfonate (DMPS) or dimercaptosuccinic acid (DMSA) can also be used to treat mercury toxicity. Once heavy-metal toxicity has been established, you should be treated by a physician experienced in chelation therapy.

Locating a Doctor Who Does Chelation Therapy

The following organizations can help you find a chelation specialist:

- ACAM
  American College of Advancement in Medicine
  24411 Ridge Route, Suite 115
  Laguna Hills, CA 92653
  (949) 309-3520
  (800) 532-3688
  http://www.acam.org

- ICIM
  International College of Integrative Medicine
  Box 271
  Bluffton, Ohio 45817
  (419) 358-0273
  www.icimed.com

How About Mercury Toxicity?

People with both lead and mercury in their bodies should be aware that these two metals have synergistic toxic effects. The presence of both metals represents a one hundredfold increase in toxicity compared to lead or mercury exposure alone. Mercury is also considered to be the most toxic substance after radioactive elements such as plutonium. In spite of this, dental mercury amalgams containing mercury are placed in the teeth of millions of Americans each year—in a location that lies between the brain and the thyroid gland.

So What Is Chelation Therapy?

The history of chelation therapy started about 100 years ago with Nobel Prize winner Alfred Werner, a Swiss chemist, who received the prize for his work on the foundation of metal-ligand binding chemistry. Metal-ligand complexes are the basis for chelation therapy. Simply put, chelation binds specific toxic metals to chelating agents. When a toxic metal binds with the chelating agent, the toxic metal is extracted from the tissues and organs of the body. Once they are bound together, the chelating agent and the toxic metal are simply excreted through the kidneys and intestinal tract.

By 1948, the United States Navy successfully used ethylene-diamine-tetra-acetic acid (EDTA) as a chelating agent for lead poisoning. One of the side benefits of EDTA chelation therapy has been dramatic improvement in arteriosclerosis. EDTA chelation therapy has also caused improvement in symptoms associated with angina, gangrene, and neuropathy. In many patients, memory, sight, and other sensory functions also improved. Many patients also report improved vitality. In addition to EDTA, there are many other chelating agents that have been developed for a variety of heavy-metal toxicities.

Chelation Therapy Is a Mystery to Most Doctors

Chelation therapy is an enigma to most of the medical community. Many medical doctors oppose the use of chelation therapy without understanding the scientific merit of the chemical function of chelating agents. Chelation therapy has provoked a lot of antagonism in mainstream medicine for its use as an alternative to bypass surgery in cardiovascular patients. For several decades, chelation has been used by alternative medical doctors to resolve conditions, such as angina with chest pain, heart attack conditions, stroke, leg cramps due to poor circulation, and poor wound healing.

EDTA chelation therapy has been approved by FDA for the removal of lead—and no other heavy metals. State medical boards are cracking down on alternative medical physicians who use chelation therapy for toxic metals other than lead—especially for the treatment of cardiovascular disease, the #1 killer in the United States.

Chelation Therapy's Other Benefits

Is there any scientific merit for chelation therapy for purposes other than reducing heavy-metal toxicity? I believe the answer is an overwhelming "Yes." The following list includes chelation therapy's other benefits:

- Reduced Cancer Deaths
  Calcium EDTA therapy reduced cancer deaths by 90% in 59 patients over 18 years. (Blumer and Reich, 1989, *Journal of Advances in Medicine*).

- Improved EKG and Exercise Capacity
  In a Danish medical study, Hancke and Flytlie reported that 69% of 253 patients had improved EKG and exercise capacity, and 58 out of 65 patients on waiting list for a heart bypass operation avoided surgery.

Chelation therapy, performed on an outpatient basis at a doctor's office, is a safe and effective treatment for heavy-metal toxicity. It is effective for many illnesses because free radicals and inflammation, caused by heavy metals, are neutralized when the heavy metals are bound and extracted from the contaminated tissues and organs.

There are many standard pharmaceutical-chelating agents available for heavy-metal toxicity in both oral and intravenous form that are available through the care of a physician. EDTA as a chelating agent has been the most well known for lead toxicity. DMPS is also a chelating agent that has been used for mercury and lead toxicity in Europe for over 50 years. Other well-known chelating agents include d-penicillamine for copper and mercury toxicity, DMSA for arsenic, lead, and mercury toxicity, and deferoxamine for iron toxicity. There are also nutritional and over-the-counter homeopathic remedies available for the general public.

Our Toxic Planet

Unfortunately, we live in a very toxic environment from which we cannot escape. Our planet has been intensively contaminated over the last 100 years. The industrial revolution started with coal burning and later switched to petrochemical-based industries. Industry and commerce have spewed vast quantities of chemicals (over 6,000 active

---

Toxic Metals in Fertilizer

In 1999, the EPA found 20 out of 29 fertilizers purchased in 12 states contained toxic metal levels that exceeded EPA limits set for waste destined to public landfills.

synthetic compounds) and heavy metals into our air, water, land, and food at an alarming rate.

Pollution is carried by air currents and rain over the entire Earth and there has been an unparalleled chemical contamination of air, water, land, and food on Earth. No one can escape pollution—even on a remote Pacific island, in a forest in Siberia, or on a barren mountain in the Andes. The FDA's warning to pregnant women is just one simple example of the damage that is being done by heavy metals. The effects of chronic mercury toxicity are subtle and cumulative. Other common heavy-metal toxicities are lead, aluminum, cadmium, nickel, tin, copper, and arsenic.

Metals Are Associated With New Emerging Illnesses

Heavy-metal toxicities have been associated with new and emerging chronic illnesses that do not fit into current medical models. Examples include chronic fatigue, fibromyalgia, attention-deficit/hyperactivity disorder (ADD/ADHD), autism, hormonal imbalance, infertility, low sex drive, depression, insomnia, anxiety, neuropathy, memory loss, irritability, moodiness, muscle weakness, cancer, unexplainable cardio-vascular problems, and many other unexplained illnesses.

Five Principles Why People Do Not Get Well

When you have been sick for a long time and you have seen many doctors without improvement of your symptoms, you should consider checking for heavy-metal toxicity. However, heavy metal toxicity is just one of five principal reasons why people are not getting well. All five that I have mentioned in articles on my Web site (www. preventionandhealing.com) include:

• Heavy-metal toxicity
• Parasites

• Food allergies
• Poor diet and nutrition
• Dental problems

Chelation therapy is only a part of the treatment plan for a chronically ill person. In every chronically ill patient I see in my practice, I always detect all five underlying causes for a chronic problem. Besides removing heavy metals, diet, nutrition, drainage remedies, dietary supplementation, and hormonal support are also part of an individualized rejuvenation program.

National Institutes of Health's TACT Study of Chelation Therapy

The National Institutes of Health (NIH) Trial to Assess Chelation Therapy (TACT) was launched in 2003 and is expected to be completed this year (2009). The 35 million dollar study is a trial of office-based, intravenous disodium ethylene-diamine-tetra-acetic acid (EDTA) as a treatment for coronary artery disease (CAD).

You don't have to wait for the NIH study. The scientific evidence for the biologic effects of the low-dose heavy-metal toxicity is overwhelming. Chelation therapy can be a new turning point for your pursuit of wellness and happiness. Or, another option would be to chelate tuna fish and clean up the Planet Earth!

Food Grown With Contaminated Fertilizer

In 2001, the *Environmental News Service* reported that food grown with contaminated fertilizer is the greatest single source of pollution exposure.

Side Effects and Symptoms From Heavy Metals

Although the body can become polluted with many different heavy metals, mercury, lead, and aluminum are the three most common metals that I see in my patients.

The following list is a summary of side effects and symptoms compiled by Analytical Research Labs, Inc. (ARL) that has been doing hair tissue analysis for three decades (www.arltma.com):

Mercury

Physical, Mental, and Neurological Symptoms
Ataxia (lack of coordinated muscle movement)
Birth defects
Dizziness
Fatigue
Hearing loss
Immune system dysfunction
Irregular heart beat
Migraine headaches
Multiple sclerosis
Numbness or tingling
Salivation (excessive)
Thyroid dysfunction
Tremors
Vision loss
Weakness (muscle)

(Mercury, Continued)

Depression
Hyperactivity
Insomnia
Irritability
Lack of concentration
Loss of self-control
Memory loss
Mood swings
Nervousness

Lead

Physical, Mental, and Neurological Symptoms
Anemia
Arthritis
Cardiovascular disease
Convulsions
Deafness
Dizziness
Encephalopathy (an acute disease of the brain)
Fatigue
Headaches
Hyperthyroidism (overactive thyroid)
Hypopituitarism (deficiency in pituitary hormone)
Impotency
Infertility
Tooth decay

(Lead, Continued)

Tremors
Confusion

Aluminum

Physical, Mental, and Neurological Symptoms

Anemia

Dental cavities

Fatigue

Headaches

Hypoparathyroidism (decreased function of the parathyroid glands, leading to decreased levels of parathyroid hormone [PTH] leading to hypocalcemia, a serious medical condition).

Kidney dysfunction

Neuromuscular dysfunction

Alzheimer's

Dementia

Mental confusion

Poor memory

Patient Testimonial
Depression and Anger Due to Mercury Toxicity

Four years ago, my husband left college with no job or insurance and three of us moved back to my hometown to rent a small house from my Mom. We also found dental care at a local college. Within 30 days of having six of my teeth treated with amalgam fillings, I became depressed, angry, and unhappy with a 6-year marriage.

(…)

It has been 3 years and we are just about complete with (mercury removal) in my mouth. It took supplements and dental work to rid my body of the mercury. The healing didn't come overnight, but I noticed changes in chunks. About every 3 or 4 months, I would think I feel better. I haven't been sick, depressed, or yelled at anyone. My energy level is high, and most of all, my husband and son have noticed an improvement.

For more of this patient's case history and testimonial, see page 337.

5

Dental
Death Trap

*One of the most important revelations of Dr. Price's
research concerned how bacteria in the teeth
act much like cancer cells that metastasize to
other parts of the body (...) where they can
infect any organ, gland, or body tissue.*

- Dr. George Meinig
Root Canal Cover Up

Your teeth and dental problems are rarely included in a
medical doctor's diagnostic assessment. If you have seen
many doctors for your condition with an unsuccessful
diagnosis, your mouth may be a missing link to your illness. Amalgams (silver fillings) and root canals are the likely causes of dental-
induced illnesses, and they are often major contributors to a wide
variety of unexplained symptoms.

Where Does Disease Really Begin?

Illness develops because one's immune system is weakened. This is
indisputable, yet often not acknowledged. Complementary and alternative medicine are based upon this premise. A disease represents a "red
flag" that a person has sustained immune system deterioration for some
time. To eliminate illness, the immune network needs to be strengthened,
yet very few people understand this principle. The box on the next page
provides a review of the components of the immune system.

What Is the Immune Network?

Your immune system comprises several organ and cell components that are easily disabled by dangerous metals commonly used in modern dental procedures. Physiological factors such as pH can also be affected by the presence of metal in the body. Components of your immune system include:

- Skin and mucous membranes
  The skin and mucous membranes of the body form a physical barrier that protects the body from foreign agents.

- pH, temperature, and oxygen
  These three physiological factors help to limit microbial growth in the body.

- Protein secretions of the body
  Several protein secretions that help limit invasion from microbial invaders including lysozyme, complement, interferon, and C-reactive protein.

- Gastrointestinal tract
  The gastrointestinal tract is one of our most important barriers of protection. Over 60 percent of our immune system is located in the intestinal lining. Specialized cells called Peyer's patches, located in the gut-associated lymphatic tissue (GALT), perform an immunological function.

- Blood and lymph systems
  The white blood cells of the body, as well as the phagocytic cells of the lymph system, defend the body against numerous pathogens and toxins.

Immune System Destroyers

Immune system destroyers that are used in dentistry include metals, principally mercury. If any of these metals begin to accumulate anywhere in your immune network, it can block the body's natural functions and form a vulnerable link in the entire immune system, creating favorable conditions for a vast range of illnesses. More often, many factors bombard the immune system over time. While symptoms are not immediately apparent, the progressive weakening of the immune system can lead to chronic illness that cannot be attributed to one specific cause.

Alternative Medicine Offers Informational Clues

Unlike most conventional medical disciplines, alternative medicine examines the whole person as a means to uncover the informational clues necessary for proper therapy. The five principal causes of immune system deterioration include:

- Heavy-metal toxicity
- Food allergies
- Dental problems (often hidden)
- Parasites
- Poor diet and nutrition

Examining the causes of an illness is not typically part of conventional medicine's approach to treatment. "Alt med," as it is often called, not only looks at the cause of disease, it also offers tools to restore the body's own immune system.

Mercury Has Been a Known Toxin Since the Mid-1800s

The most dangerous metal that is used in dentistry is mercury. Even though mercury has been a known toxin since the mid-1800s, the

American Dental Association maintains that, in the composition of the amalgam alloy, mercury is nontoxic. There is actually a significant amount of mercury in a silver filling, and there is also evidence that it spreads to the rest of the body:

- **Mercury Content in Amalgam Fillings**
  The silver in amalgam fillings contains 50 percent mercury, 20 to 30 percent silver, as well as trace amounts of tin, copper, and zinc.

- **Study That Shows Mercury Spreads**
  Studies have proven that mercury from fillings spreads through the entire body. A University of Calgary Medical School study on sheep followed the path of mercury through the sheeps' bodies and discovered that within 28 or 29 days, mercury had spread throughout the animals' entire bodies, including crossing the placental barrier. The researchers discovered that mercury that had spread was massively concentrated in the intestinal area.

Dental Amalgam Is Considered to be a Toxic Waste

Most people do not realize that the Environmental Protection Agency (EPA) considers mercury to be a toxic waste. Dr. Ron Kennedy, who wrote an article called "Dental Amalgam Mercury Poisoning," provides details of the EPA's policy concerning the handling of mercury after it leaves a patient's mouth (See: www.savvypatients.com/amalgam.htm).

The federal agency responsible for regulation of allowable levels of substances at the workplace has established 50 μg/cc (μg = micrograms) as the maximum allowable level of mercury vapor in the workplace. The average level of mercury vapor in the mouths of people with amalgams varies between 50 and 150 μg/cc. When removed from your mouth, dental amalgam is considered a toxic waste by the Environmental Protection Agency and must be handled in a certain way to protect dental office personnel from mercury poisoning. This is the same stuff, unchanged, which just came out of your tooth! There are over 125 known symptoms of mercury toxicity.

Root Canals Are Another Major Source of Illness

A root canal, very simply, is the removal of the material in the middle of the tooth and down into the root of the tooth, in order to remove an infection (See: "What Is a Root Canal Procedure?"). The problem with a root canal is that, although its purpose is to remove an immediate infection, the procedure itself leads to further chronic infection over time. Dr. Weston A. Price (1870-1948), a renowned dental specialist, determined that many types of degenerative diseases were caused by root canals. These include many forms of heart disease, kidney and bladder diseases, arthritis, rheumatism, mental diseases, lung diseases, and many forms of cancer. Price was the the chairman of, and a leading researcher for, the research section of the American Dental Association from 1914 to 1923. In 1923, he published a two-volume work of 1174 pages detailing his findings on the danger of root canals and old tooth extraction sites. His work also described associated infections, as well as the systemic effect on the body. Dr. Price's work on root canals is summarized in a book called *Root Canal Cover Up* by Dr. George Meinig, D.D.S. (See: Dr. George Meinig's *Root Canal Cover Up*).

Repairing Dental Problems

Dental problems may be repaired by replacing amalgams with non-metal materials and correcting root canals. This requires a financial commitment, patience, and persistence. Correcting dental problems is one major step toward reaping the rewards of eliminating chronic illness and restoring vigor to one's health. Biological dentists understand the dangers of modern dentistry, and they play a vital role in

How to Find a Biological Dentist

The International Academy of Oral Medicine and Toxicology (IAOMT) believes that it is not possible to create a "safe" mercury amalgam, and the dentists in the IOAMT network practice a biological approach to dentistry. Their Web site contains a look-up feature that may be used to locate biological dentists across the country (www.iaomt.org).

IAOMT email: info@iaomt.org
Phone: (863) 420-6373
Fax: (863) 419-8136 24 hours
Mon. through Fri. 10:00 AM to 4:00 PM
Eastern Standard Time

International Academy of Biological Dentistry and Medicine
19122 Camelia Bend Circle
Spring, Texas 77379
(281) 651-1785
www.iabdm.org

Note: For a list of St. Louis biological dentists, see page 426.

the recovery from dental-induced chronic illness. This unique group of dentists work closely with alternative medical doctors who understand the importance of the dental-body connection. As a team, these practitioners look at the whole person to understand the root cause of illness.

Connection Between Oral Bacteria and Disease

The subject of the connection between degenerative diseases and oral bacteria that can become entrenched inside teeth is surprisingly complex because it relates to several interrelated factors including:

- Hidden dental infections caused by root canal procedures or an infected cavitation from an improperly extracted tooth (usually a wisdom tooth)

- A decline in the immune system due to inadequate nutrition

- A taxed immune system that is overwhelmed by:

  - Immune-destroying chemicals in food and water

  - Heavy metals

  - Bacteria and other microorganisms in food and water

- Blockages in the body's biocybernetic matrix that leads to signaling errors and altered tissue states

  Understanding these issues is half the battle. We will first explore some background details and then present practical strategies that you can use to help your immune system eliminate any invading bacteria.

What Is a Root Canal Procedure?

Root canal therapy, which consists of filling in the root canal in the tooth, often leaves bacteria in the dentin tubules and surrounding area. There are approximately three miles of micron-sized dentin tubules in most teeth.

A root canal is the main canal within the dentin of the tooth. Human teeth have one to four canals containing connective tissue referred to as dental pulp. The canal in each tooth is anatomically connected to other canals in other teeth, and blood vessels inside millions of microscopic tubules in the dental pulp supply nutrition to the teeth. When the dental pulp inside a tooth is infected, there is a risk that the infection will spread to other teeth or to the jaw. Although root canal therapy is a widely accepted endodontic procedure (30 million root

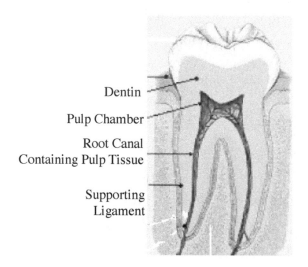

Dentin

Pulp Chamber

Root Canal
Containing Pulp Tissue

Supporting
Ligament

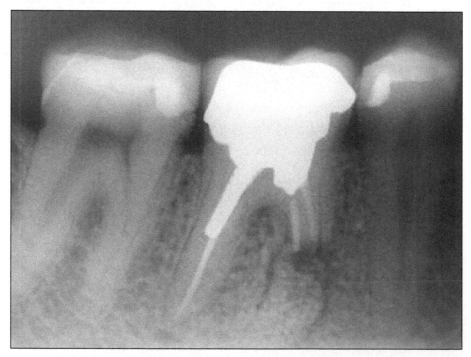

Figure: X-ray image of a tooth that has had a root canal procedure.

canals are filled annually), it is increasingly viewed as a controversial procedure ever since a founding member of the American Association of Endodontists published a book that says root canals cause degenerative diseases (See: Dr. George Meinig's *Root Canal Cover Up*). Here is a timeline that will help readers understand the root canal controversy:

- During the early part of the 20th century, a popular "focal infection theory" said it is impossible to clean out (and fill) the millions of microscopic tubules in the tooth's dentin. Once inside these tubules, bacteria can grow and multiply, transforming themselves into anaerobic organisms that need less oxygen.

  Note: Focal infection simply means that an infection in one part of the body travels to, and creates an infection in, another part of the body. In the early 1900s, prominent doctors around the country published research demonstrating that germs from a walled-off area (such as a root canal or cavitation resulting from an incompletely extracted tooth) can metastasize to other organs and tissues. Today, it is openly accepted that dental infection can cause endocarditis (an infection of the heart valves) and rheumatic heart disease. It is also known and accepted that individuals with joint replacements, such as a hip replacement, must take antibiotics before every dental visit due to the spreading of bacteria from the teeth to the joints. Dental focal infection is very serious, and it covers all aspects of chronic degenerative medical conditions. This includes arthritis, cancer, neurological disorders, and many other conditions too numerous to mention.

- During this same period (the early 20th century), a dentist named Dr. Weston A. Price devoted 25 years to the investigation of focal infection. His research, involving thousands of patients and rabbits, proved that focal infections cause systemic disease.

Pleomorphism of Bacteria

Another aspect of dental infections that is truly remarkable involves the pleomorphic ability of bacteria. Under the right conditions, cells, particularly one-celled organisms, can change into cells of another type. Cells that adapt and mutate in extreme environmental conditions can make infections reappear years later. Pathogenic microorganisms can change shape and size, thrive in the absence of oxygen, and become stronger—with their toxins becoming more toxic. In view of this, it is important to understand that long-term antibiotic therapies only promote prolific mutation and pleomorphism.

- After World War II, antibiotics, x-rays, and anesthetics popularized an endodontic procedure called root canal therapy. The procedure involves a sterilization procedure designed to clean and seal the larger infected pulp tubules to prevent contamination of the entire root canal system (See figure, page 86).

- The focal infection theory receded for several decades until 1993 when Dr. George Meinig self-published his *Root Canal Cover Up*. Around this same time, biological dentistry emerged—emphasizing a relationship between oral and systemic health.

Modern endodontists who perform root canal procedures believe that antibiotics and the body's immune system are able to neutralize any trapped bacteria in microscopic tubules. However, early twentieth century dentists, including Dr. Weston A. Price, knew otherwise.

What Is a Cavitation?

A cavitation is a cavity within a jawbone that previously held a tooth. It is a socket of an old tooth extraction site that has not filled in completely. A cavitation infection is a silent jawbone condition that occurs when a remaining periodontal membrane in the bony socket gets infected. This leaves spaces in the bone of the jaw that allows infections to grow. Cavitation infection (infection in the bony socket of the tooth and jaw bone) can be infected with 20 to 30 different species of bacteria. Lab results often reveal a condition known as ischemic osteonecrosis or bone death due to poor delivery of oxygen or blood supply to a local area.

To prevent this type of infection from occurring, a dentist who does an extraction needs to remove the periodontal ligament or membrane that holds the tooth in the socket.

Wisdom Teeth Are Extracted From Most American Teenagers

Wisdom tooth extractions or other teeth are part of a ritual of most American teenagers as they become adults in the United States. What is unknown and shocking is that tooth socket infections are very common after tooth extractions. These infections are often overlooked as the cause of unexplained symptoms from fatigue, headaches, arthritic pain, heart problems, insomnia, neurological symptoms, hormone imbalance, emotional and psychological disturbances, intestinal problems, and severe facial pain.

The time it takes for medical symptoms to occur after a tooth extraction can vary from a few weeks to many years. The time depends on a person's general physical condition, nutritional state, and adaptability to stress. Whenever young people develop unexplainable medical symptoms, I immediately think of an old, infected wisdom tooth socket.

Cavitations Are Overlooked and Untreated

The lack of a reliable test for cavitations and the fact that tooth extractions cause minimal dental discomfort has allowed cavitations to be almost entirely overlooked and untreated. As a result, cavitations are very rarely suspected as a cause of a chronic medical problem. Kinesiology muscle testing, bone scans, and thermographic imaging have all been used to localize and identify dental problems, but none of these have been consistently reliable.

Identifying Hidden Dental Infections

Acupuncture Meridian Assessment, which I have described elsewhere in this book, is a new way of assessing our body energy flows based on acupuncture principles. This technology can guide a qualified practitioner to find hidden cavitations and other dental infections. Complex dental-medical patterns are often seen in patients who have been previously evaluated by numerous medical specialists with unsuccessful results. Besides hidden dental problems, the other common causes of complex medical problems are parasites, food allergies, heavy-metal problems, and nutritional deficiencies. When dental infections are properly corrected, the response can be almost miraculous.

As this point, you're probably wondering, "If infections from root canals are so common, and such a frequent cause of many unexplained medical symptoms, why is this not commonly known among the dental and medical professions?" The answer to this question is revealed in a 70-year cover-up that is explained in Dr. George E. Meinig's book, *Root Canal Cover Up* (See: Dr. George Meinig's *Root Canal Cover Up*).

The Body's Biocybernetic Matrix and Its Connection to Teeth

Few Americans realize that while cellular biochemistry and genes are the primary focus of Western allopathic medicine, researchers on the cutting edge of alternative medicine (in Germany and Asia) are exploring energy and information phenomena in the body's internal environment (otherwise known as the "terrain").

In the 1940s, an Austrian physician named Alfred Pischinger challenged the Louis Pasteur germ theory of disease that was promoted in the mid-19th century. Pischinger and a team of researchers proved scientifically that it is not a single germ that causes disease but a set of conditions that are part of a regulatory *system* (See also: "What is Biological Terrain Analysis and Who Was Professor Louis Claude Vincent?"). In the last 20 years, Professor and Doctor of Natural Sciences Hartmut Heine and his colleagues have carried on Pischinger's work. They refer to a "matrix" (also known as a "ground," "milieu," or "biological terrain") in the body that "pervades extracellular space and reaches every cell in the body." The following points summarize important concepts about the body's internal matrix or terrain:

- Every function and every process is related to the matrix in some form.

- Every cell is nourished through the matrix.

- All waste products of cellular metabolism pass through the matrix.

- All immune response and tissue repair take place in the matrix.

- The matrix is not an inert filler substance but a body-wide communication and support system.

- Recent research has shown that the matrix comprises semiconducting liquid crystals that have properties for the transmission, storage, and processing of information.

Metal in the Mouth Creates a Battery

When two dissimilar metals are used in fillings or crowns, they produce current due to a phenomena known as electrogalvanism. Electrical current that is produced in the mouth has detrimental side effects including:

- **Toxic metal release**
  Toxic metals are released from dental metals, even without current, but two or more dissimilar metals cause additional leaching.

- **Brain and nervous system dysfunction**
  The nervous system is inherently electrical and the current produced by dental metals causes disturbances in the body's nervous system.

  Indirectly, a disturbance to the brain and nervous system can cause problems such as allergies, chronic fatigue, psychiatric and endocrine disorders, gastrointestinal problems, multiple sclerosis (MS), neuropathy, amyotrophic lateral sclerosis (ALS), also known as Lou Gehrig's Disease, osteoporosis, reproductive problems, kidney disease, heart disease (especially arrhythmia, electrical dysfunction, or bacterial disease), high blood pressure, lung and respiratory problems, skin disease, as well as birth defects.

Search for a Dentist Who Understands Galvanic Current
Galvanic current is so detrimental that it is imperative that you search for a dentist who understands the consequences of mixing metals in the mouth. Dentists have been using dissimilar metals in dental procedures for over 100 years, and electrogalvanism is not a topic that is taught in dental schools. All holistic dentists are self-taught, and there

are very few good dentists. Most are swayed by conventional medicine. Electrogalvanism may be a topic that you can
use to help select a dentist.

- The human body depends on the matrix for its health, because
  it reacts to every toxic irritation that we are bombarded with
  (pathogens, chemicals, malnutrition).
- The sum of the toxic irritations in the matrix can lead to exhaustion due to energy blockages along the body's energy meridians,
  making the body more vulnerable to disease.

Kramer, Voll, and the Link to Teeth

In mid-20th century Germany, research conducted by a dentist
named Dr. Fritz Kramer and a medical doctor named Dr. Reinhold
Voll helped doctors and dentists (mostly in Germany) understand the
relationship between local infections in the mouth and distant illness
elsewhere in the body. Here are their contributions:

- **Dr. Fritz Kramer**
  Kramer mapped the relationship between the teeth and organs
  of the body (See: tooth-organ charts in this chapter).

- **Dr. Reinhold Voll**
  Voll developed an electroacupuncture device for measuring
  electrical potential at the body's acupuncture points. He was
  able to demonstrate that electrical changes in acupuncture points
  are related to disease conditions in the body. He also demonstrated that a local infection in the mouth can disrupt the energy
  flow along the body's meridians and negatively affect the
  body's terrain.

Energetic Relationship Between Teeth and Organs of the Body

The energetic relationship that Kramer and Voll discovered between teeth and organs of the body are due to the body's meridians that are defined in Traditional Chinese medicine. Every tooth crosses one or more of the body's 12 major meridians. The following diagrams will help readers understand the meridian relationships between the teeth and organs:

- **Kidney and Bladder Meridians**
  A disturbance in the teeth that touches your kidney and bladder meridians can affect these two organs, as well as your urogenital tract. A disturbance can also affect the ankles, rectum, and anal canal, nose, the frontal sinus, and the adrenal and pineal glands.

Kidney and Bladder Meridian

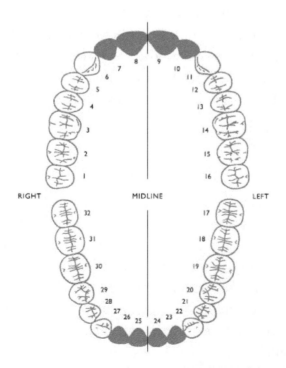

- **Liver and Gallbladder Meridians**
  A disturbance in the teeth that touches your liver and gallbladder meridians can affect these organs, as well as the sphenoidal sinus, hips, gonads, and pituitary gland.

Liver and Gallbladder Meridian

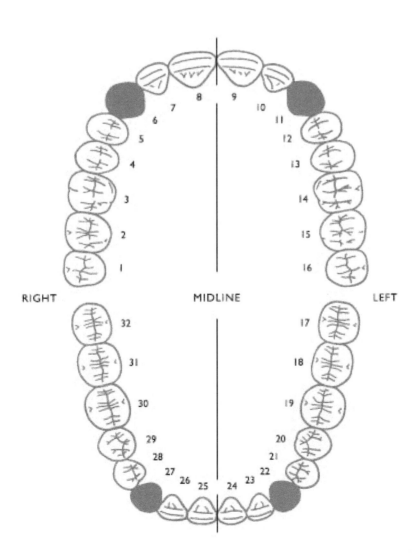

- **Large Intestine and Lung Meridians**
  A disturbance in the teeth that touches the large intestine and lung meridians can affect these organs, as well as small intestine, lungs, veins, arteries, hands, feet, nose, shoulders, or the pituitary or thymus glands.

Large Intestine and Lung Meridian

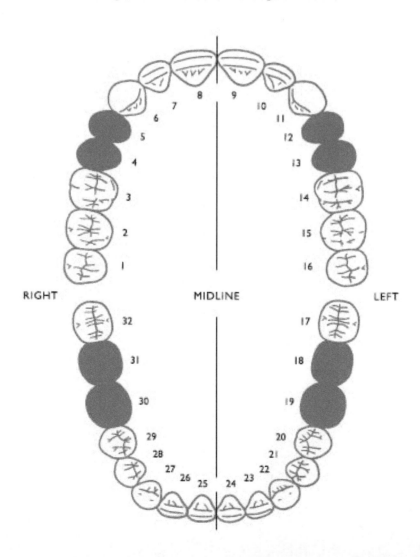

- **Stomach and Spleen Meridians**

  A disturbance in the teeth that touches the stomach and spleen
  meridians can affect these organs, as well as the pancreas,
  esophagus, parathyroid gland, mammary glands, stomach, knee
  and ankle joints, lymph vessels, maxillary sinuses, or the thyroid
  gland.

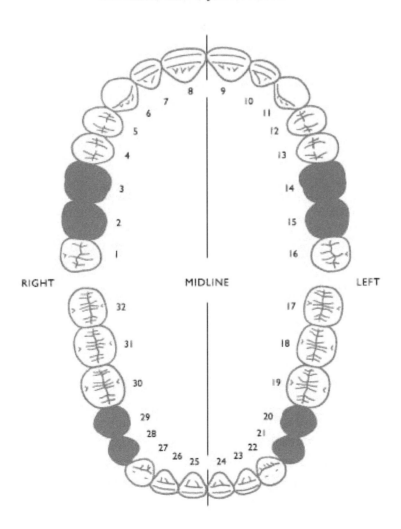

Stomach and Spleen Meridian

- **Heart, Small Intestine, Triple Warmer,
  and Circulation/Sex Meridians**
  A disturbance in the teeth that touches these meridians will affect
  the heart, small intestine, and nervous system, as well as the
  shoulders, elbows, hands, feet, ears, tongue, sacroiliac joint, and
  limbic system.

Heart, Small Intestine, Triple Warmer, and
Circulation/Sex Meridians

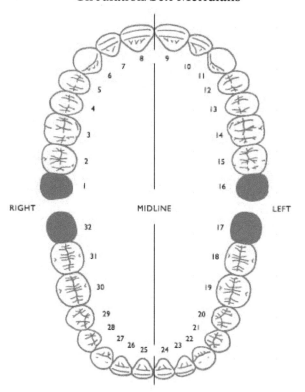

The Tooth-Organ Meridian chart on the next page further illustrates
how the mouth and the body are connected. What affects a person's
teeth can affect an organ (or organs) in the same body.

Tooth-Organ Meridian Chart

Upper Teeth

	1	2	3	4	5	6	7	8	9	10	11	12	13	14	15	16
Sense Organs	Inner ear	Maxillary sinus		Ethmoid cells	Eye	Frontal sinus			Frontal sinus			Eye	Ethmoid cells	Maxillary sinus		Inner ear
Joints	Shoulder, Elbow / Hand, ulnar Foot, plantar Toes, sacro-iliac joint	Jaws / Front of knee		Shoulder, Elbow / Hand, radial Foot Big toe	Hip	Back of knee / Sacrococcyx / Foot			Back of knee / Sacrococcyx / Foot			Hip	Shoulder, Elbow / Hand, radial Foot Big toe	Jaws / Front of knee		Shoulder, Elbow / Hand, ulnar Foot, plantar Toes, sacro-iliac joint
Spinal Segments	C8 T1 T5 T6 T7 S1 S2 S3	T11 T12 L1		C5 C6 C7 T2 T3 T4 L4 L5	T8 T9 T10	L2 L3 S4 S5 Coccyx			L2 L3 S4 S5 Coccyx			T8 T9 T10	C5 C6 C7 T2 T3 T4 L4 L5	T11 T12 L1		C8 T1 T5 T6 T7 S1 S2 S3
Vertebrae	C7 T1 T5 T6 S1 S2	T11 T12 L1		C5 C6 C7 T2 T3 T4 L4 L5	T9 T10	L2 L3 S3 S4 S5 Coccyx			L2 L3 S3 S4 S5 Coccyx			T9 T10	C5 C6 C7 T2 T3 T4 L4 L5	T11 T12 L1		C7 T1 T5 T6 S1 S2
Organs	Heart-R / Duodenum	Pancreas / Stomach-R		Lung-R / Large Intestine-R	Liver-R / Gall-blad-der	Kidney-R / Bladder-R Urogenital area			Kidney-L / Bladder-L Urogenital area			Liver-L / Bile ducts -L	Lung-L / Large Intestine-L	Spleen / Stomach-L		Heart-L / Jejunum Ileum-L
Endocrine Organs	Pituitary, Ant. lobe	Para-thyroid	Thy-roid	Thy-mus	Pituitary, Post lobe	Pineal gland			Pineal gland			Pituitary, Post lobe	Thy-mus	Thy-roid	Para-thyroid	Pituitary, Ant. lobe
Others	CNS Psyche	Mammary Gland-R												Mammary Gland-L		CNS Psyche
Upper Teeth	R — 1	2	3	4	5	6	7	8	9	10	11	12	13	14	15	16 — L

Lower Teeth

	32	31	30	29	28	27	26	25	24	23	22	21	20	19	18	17
Lower Teeth	R — 32	31	30	29	28	27	26	25	24	23	22	21	20	19	18	17 — L
Others	Energy Metabolism		Mammary Gland-R											Mammary Gland-L		Energy Metabolism
Endocrine Glands Tissue System	Peripheral nerves	Ar-teries	Veins	Lymph vessels	Gonad (Testes or Overy)	Adrenal gland			Adrenal gland			Gonad (Testes or Overy)	Lymph vessels	Veins	Ar-teries	Peripheral nervous system
Organs	Ileum-R / Heart-R	Large Intestine-R (Ileoceal region) / Lung-R		Stomach-R Pylorus / Pancreas	Gall-blad-der / Liver-R	Bladder-R Urogenital area / Kidney-R			Bladder-L Urogenital area / Kidney-L			Bile ducts -L / Liver-L	Stomach-L / Spleen	Large Intestine-L / Lung-L		Jejunum Ileum-L / Heart-L
Vertebrae	C7 T1 T5 T6 S1 S2	C5 C6 C7 T2 T3 T4 L4 L5		T11 T12 L1	T9 T10	L2 L3 S3 S4 S5 Coccyx			L2 L3 S3 S4 S5 Coccyx			T9 T10	T11 T12 L1	C5 C6 C7 T2 T3 T4 L4 L5		C7 T1 T5 T6 S1 S2
Spinal Segments	C8 T1 T5 T6 T7 S1 S2 S3	C5 C6 C7 T2 T3 T4 L4 L5		T11 T12 L1	T8 T9 T10	L2 L3 S4 S5 Coccyx			L2 L3 S4 S5 Coccyx			T8 T9 T10	T11 T12 L1	C5 C6 C7 T2 T3 T4 L4 L5		C8 T1 T5 T6 T7 S1 S2 S3
Joints	Shoulder and elbow / Hand, ulnar Foot, plantar Toes, sacro-iliac joint	Front of knee / Hand, radial Foot Big toe		Hip / Jaws	Sacrococcyx / Foot	Back of knee / Foot			Back of knee / Foot			Sacrococcyx / Foot	Hip / Jaws	Front of knee / Hand, radial Foot Big toe		Shoulder and elbow / Hand, ulnar Foot, plantar Toes, sacro-iliac joint
Sense Organs	Ear	Ethmoid cells		Maxillary Sinus	Eye	Frotal sinus			Frotal sinus			Eye	Maxillary Sinus	Ethmoid cells		Ear

Prevention and Healing, Inc. by Simon Yu, M.D., (314) 432-7802. *Note: A scalable version of this chart is available in color on my Web site at www.preventionandhealing.com.*

What Is Biological Terrain Analysis (BTA) and Who Was Professor Louis Claude Vincent?

Biological terrain analysis (BTA) is the evaluation of body fluids to assess the condition of the matrix (or terrain).

In the 1930s, a French hydrologist named Professor Louis-Claude Vincent became interested in measuring parameters reflective of human health and created a system known as the Bio Electronique Vincent. In an address at the International Convention for Medical Electronics in 1959, Vincent told his colleagues that the key to understanding health was through monitoring and controlling the body's building blocks that are found in the body fluids:

- **pH (Acid/Alkaline Balance)**
  Digestion, absorption of nutrients, activation of enzymes, binding of hormones at receptor sites, and many other biological processes are pH dependent.

- **Oxidation Reduction Potential (ORP)**
  ORP reflects the level of electrons in the biological fluid and provides an indication of energy production as well as free radical activity.

- **Resistivity**
  Resistivity refers to the electrolyte/mineral levels in the body. If fluids become congested with too many minerals (or salts), sluggish cell function issues can develop. If there are too few minerals, demineralization can occur, impacting enzyme activation, bone, and muscle development.

Dr. George Meinig's Root Canal Cover Up

Remarkably, in 1993, Dr. George Meinig, D.D.S. (1914-2008), one of the founding members of the American Association of Endodontists (root canal therapists), wrote a book called *Root Canal Cover-Up* that explains how root canals can damage health and cripple the immune system. Meinig's book is a review of Dr. Weston Price's 25 years of root canal research that was published in 1923, but buried for 70 years.

Although Meinig had been a director of the Price Pottenger Nutrition Foundation (PPNF) for 20 years, Meinig and others at the foundation had never seen Dr. Price's two books on dental infections.

Note: The Foundation's main purpose was to make Price's *Nutrition and Physical Degeneration* available to the professionals and the public.

In 1992, Dr. Hal Huggins, a controversial dentist who has published several books about the dangers of mercury amalgams, played a role in the discovery of Price's two "other books." Huggins met a friend of Price's who gave him Price's *Dental Infections, Oral and Systemic* (703 pages) and *Dental Infections and the Degenerative Diseases* (471 pages). Huggins read the books, said he could not put them down, and later delivered them to the PPNF. In a chapter in Meinig's book titled, "Alarming Cover-up of Vital Root-Canal Research Discovered," Meinig says that pressure built up for him to accept the responsibility for alerting the public about the implications of Price's research and that he finally "bit the bullet" and wrote a book that contradicts medical research's search for single organisms that cause single diseases. Price found at least 20 different organisms that were responsible for infections in teeth and his most important discovery that is still largely covered up:

Germs infecting the teeth are responsible for an enormous number of diseases that manifest in other parts of the body.

Meinig said he intended to "deliver the message about the serious side effects of root canal therapy by radio and television appearances, articles in magazines, and by lectures." Even though Dr. Meinig's book never received the kind of publicity that he hoped that it would, the PPNF reports that his self-published book has had eight printings and was recently contracted to be printed in Japanese by the Koushikai, PPNF's sister organization. By preserving a record of Dr. Weston Price's root canal research, Dr. Meinig helped to save the lives of thousands of people. Today, Meinig's book is available at Amazon.com and at the Price Pottenger Nutrition Foundation (www.ppnf.org).

Proprioception and Its Connection to Dentistry

Proprioception may be defined *as an unconscious perception of stimuli relating to the body's own position, posture, equilibrium, or internal condition.* Proprioception has been referred to as the body's sixth sense. It is part of the nervous system—but an unconscious part. An example of a proprioception mechanism is the constant gathering of sensory input that provides the body with information needed to maintain balance. A proprioception mechanism in the brain and nervous system, along with a fluid-filled network within the inner ear, helps the body orient to the pull of gravity.

Fifty years ago, neurologists were aware that the nerves in the oral cavity play an important role in the body's proprioception mechanism. There were prominent neurologists who wrote about proprioception for medical school textbooks, but much of this information has been lost. Factors that can harm this very important part of the nervous system include:

- A misaligned upper and lower jaw resulting from malnutrition or bottle feeding an infant

- Orthodontic adjustment that causes a misaligned upper and lower jaw

- A temporomandibular joint (TMJ) problem related to the jaw joint connecting the lower jaw (mandible) to the skull (temporal bone) in front of the ear.

In his book, *Energy Transcendence*, Dr. Larry Lytle quotes neurologists, Drs. Wilder Penfield and Theodore Rasmussen, who wrote *Cerebral Cortex of Man* (Macmillan, 1950):

Over 50% of the brain is devoted to the dental area.

Lytle says that Penfield and Rasmussen traced the nerves from the brain to the oral cavity. Lytle also explains mandibular/maxillary (upper jaw-lower jaw) relationship affects over 50 percent of body functions, including motor and sensory actions, blood supply to the brain, as well as low-level electrical feedback from the body to the brain.

Lytle's book, as well as a video that he recorded about proprioception makes the following connections between the nerves in the oral cavity and health:

- Proprioception is the method of feedback that causes the body or the brain to respond to messages from the rest of the body.

- The way the lower jaw fits the skull is the most important factor that affects a person's general health.

- The nerve that comes from the lower jaw, called the mandibular nerve, is the only nerve that is both motor and sensory — it gathers information and provides response messages to which the body reacts. The mandibular nerve also has fibers connected to the vagus nerve that controls all the organs of the body.

- Over 2,000 years ago, the Chinese explained that the 12 meridians of the body are controlled by areas in the oral cavity. He says that holistic dentists make a mistake by assuming that this refers to the teeth. Lytle says it is not the teeth but the tightness of the muscles that control the lower jaw's connection to the skull. If these muscles are too tight, the body will have an over responsive sympathetic autonomic nervous system (stress, malfuntioning organs) and an underresponsive parasympathetic autonomic nervous system.

- Lytle says that the autonomic nervous system, with its sympathetic and parasympathetic branches, controls overall health. Lytle's solution is a light laser that may be applied to the muscles of the jaw to balance these two systems.

Chapter's Important Conclusion: Think Dental

An important conclusion to draw from the information presented in this chapter:

> *When the latest medical therapy fails, think dental.*
> *(Your dental problems can be your death trap!*
> *Choose your dentist very carefully.)*

Patient Success Story
Breast Cancer and Mercury Removal

If I were to tell "my story'"to a group of cancer patients and offer them a checklist of what is essential to do to heal yourself, removing heavy metals (mercury) would be top on the list.

For more of this patient's case history and success story,
see page 292.

Notes

6

Fighting the Body's Invaders: Parasites

Deep knowledge is to be aware of disturbance before disturbance, to be aware of danger before danger, to be aware of destruction before destruction, to be aware of calamity before calamity.

Sun Tzu
The Art of War
China, 500 B.C.

In March 2005, *Science* magazine published a special issue called "Stealth Invaders: Parasites and Pathogens." In a military context, the word "stealth" is often used to describe a hidden invader:

…the act or action of proceeding furtively, secretly, or imperceptibly

The magazine's use of the word "stealth" is appropriate because the body is routinely invaded by invisible parasites that range in size from small single-celled organisms to larger parasitic worms that usually enter the body as eggs. This chapter describes how I first discovered parasites, and it also contains some self-help strategies for dealing with invaders.

The Bolivia Connection: The U.S. Army Targets Parasites

My new patients always ask me with a certain skepticism why I use parasite medications for their conditions when no other doctors seem concerned about parasites. Most American medical doctors hardly have any experience with parasites or any experience using parasite medications. My story starts with my experience in Bolivia while serving as a U.S. Army Reserve Medical Officer.

American Peace-Keeping Mission in Oruro

In April 2001 our U.S. Army reserve unit, 21st General Hospital from St. Louis, was assigned to Bolivia for a peace-keeping mission. Our small medical team, consisting of two medical doctors, one dentist, one veterinarian, nursing staff, and the support team flew to La Paz, Bolivia from Miami, Florida. In Bolivia, our group joined a medical group from the 2nd Division of the Bolivian Army in Oruro.

Oruro was a silver and tin mining town around 150 years ago at which time it was one of the richest cities in the world. You would never guess that fact when I was there. In 2001, Oruro was an abandoned mining town in the middle of a semi-desert in an Andes plateau.

Controversial Coca Eradication

In Bolivia, coca (not cocaine) has been consumed for thousands of years to relieve hunger, fatigue, and headaches, which are symptoms of altitude sickness. Unfortunately for poor farmers, coca plants are also used in the manufacture of cocaine. There have been many unhappy Bolivian Andes Indian farmers whose coca plants have been destroyed by the Bolivian government due to pressure from the U.S. government. The result has been an uprising and protest all over the country. Our assignment was to provide free medical care and to *please the crowds*. Our mission included preventive medical and dental care for indigenous Andes Indians as well as veterinary care for their animals.

Our Mini Medical Camp

Every morning, a Bolivian Army bus with our U.S. government-issued medical supplies took our group to small towns within a 2- to 3-hour drive and set up a mini medical camp, usually at a local school. We always had a translator who understood the local Andes dialect and could translate from Spanish to English.

Before our medical group arrived in the Bolivian towns, there would be hundreds of Andes Indians lined up waiting for free medical and dental care. We had to see them at a rate much faster than your typical HMO-managed care facility. Within the space of 2 weeks, we saw approximately 10,000 Andes Indians. As a part of the program, the majority were treated with parasite medications, either pyrantel pamoate or mebendazole, two of the most widely available inexpensive parasite medications available from the U.S. government.

The key part of my story occurred within days after the first group of Indians was treated with antiparasite medications. Several patients returned to relay stories of seeing parasites passing in their stools and a few had parasites erupt from their skin. Their stories, the samples they brought in jars, and their descriptions of how much better they were feeling left me with what later turned out to be an important question: How much chronic illness is due to parasite infection?

Parasites Are Not Part of Medical Training

I don't remember using parasite medications in my medical training or any experiences treating medical conditions related to parasite infestations. Parasites as a potential medical problem in America simply are not part of our medical training, except for the brief facts that doctors memorize for medical board exams. I do recollect a few suspicious cases of parasite problems early in my medical practice but stool tests were all negative and the patients were never treated. Why are parasite problems overlooked? First, most of the parasites have very complex life cycles that are often outside of the intestinal tract. Second, we only look at stool samples. Third, stool samples are old and semi-destroyed when collected and sent to the lab. Stool samples should be fresh. Fourth, most laboratory technicians and pathologists don't have enough training to recognize ova and parasites in the stool.

Bolivia Influenced My American Medical Practice

Since my first-hand experience in Bolivia, I've used parasite medications in various combinations. I've observed dramatic responses in my patients in situations where specialists' treatments had failed. Some of the difficult conditions that responded with parasite medications included: intractable allergies and asthma, migraine headache, sciatica, constipation and diarrhea, irritable bowel syndrome, colitis, bronchiectasis, vision loss, anxiety, depression, nightmares, TMJ (temporomandibular joint) problems, chronic fatigue, fibromyalgia, multiple sclerosis, arthralgia and myalgia, pelvic pain, eczema, psoriasis, hypertension, and others.

Electronic Signals Suggest Parasite-Like Activity

My treatment plan for parasites is based on a clinical suspicion about common symptoms that don't respond to traditional medical treatment as mentioned above. Also, I use technology based on acupuncture and Acupuncture Meridian Assessment. I've written several articles regarding Acupuncture Meridian Assessment and parasites related to medical conditions (available on www.preventionandhealing.com). I can pick up electronic signals suggesting parasitic-like activity and treat accordingly with herbal, homeopathic, and pre-scribed parasite medications.

Patient response varies depending on individual cases. Most of these patients have already been to many specialists and well-known medi-cal institutions in the country. It's hard for me to believe that parasites play such a large role in hidden causes of modern illnesses, and this hasn't been addressed and taught by the academic medical com-munity. Whenever a cause of an illness is "unknown," the medical community is quick to blame viruses. It is not viruses—it is parasites. Surprisingly, parasites are often carriers of viruses. We desperately need a better biometric technology like Acupuncture Meridian Assessment to detect and treat parasites than current teachings from schools of medicine.

Other Related and Overlooked Areas

Other overlooked causes of modern illnesses include heavy-metal toxicity, hidden dental problems, nutritional deficiency, food aller-gies, environmental toxicity, and detoxification needs. I hope I am not repeating myself, but these neglected problems often promote more susceptible medical conditions in which parasites thrive. Therefore, treating parasites is not good enough. You must correct the under-lying problems and restore the biological terrain and the immune system. Otherwise, parasites will return and repeat their complicated life cycles and baffle medical doctors. Most of the Andes Indians we treated will be reinfected in a short time through their water supply, foods, and sanitation conditions.

Many Incurable Conditions Are Related to Hidden Parasites

Without my experience in Bolivia while serving in the U.S. Army Reserve and my experience with Acupuncture Meridian Assessment, I would never have uncovered the hidden role of parasite infections.

Operation Enduring Freedom: Saving Colonel H.

An article I wrote about my experience at the Landstuhl U.S. Army Hospital in Germany during Operation Enduring Freedom in 2005 fits into this chapter.

୭ଈ ୭ଈ ୭ଈ

U.S. Army military medicine provides some of the best trauma care in the world. Wounded soldiers get immediate trauma care by well-trained field medics in the battle field. They are transferred, usually by helicopter, to a combat support hospital for surgical care, and they're stabilized by some of the best medical and surgical teams.

When stable enough to move, soldiers from Iraq and Afghanistan are air-evacuated to Ramstein Air Force Base in Germany. They are then stabilized at Landstuhl U.S. Army Hospital before returning home to the U.S. or, heading back to the battlefield.

I am retired as a Colonel in the U.S. Army Reserves after 25 years of service. I have never been on a battlefield in Iraq or Afghanistan. When I was mobilized and deployed for Operation Enduring Freedom in 2005, I was stationed at Landstuhl U.S. Army Hospital in Germany.

As an internist, I took care of active duty soldiers, civilian contractors, dependents, and evacuated soldiers from Iraq and Afghanistan for medical-related problems. Most of the trauma cases go directly to a surgical intensive care unit under the care of trauma surgeons.

Internal medicine and family practice take care of most medical-related problems. The U. S. Army has a 2-week medical evacuation policy. If a soldier cannot be medically evaluated and recover in 2 weeks, a soldier is returned to an Army Hospital in the U.S. If they can recover in 2 weeks, they return to duty in Iraq or Afghanistan.

When I was called for active duty, I took my small portable Acupuncture Meridian Assessment instrument (also called EAV for electroacupuncture according to Voll) to test patients with complicated symptoms and puzzling complaints.

My first patient at the Landstuhl Hospital was a 22-year-old Army Corporal from Missouri with undiagnosed abdominal pain that he had for 3 weeks. Extensive medical evaluation was done including a computed tomography (CT) scan at the Combat Support Hospital in Baghdad. He was then evacuated to Landstuhl U.S. Army Hospital for further evaluation.

My EAV testing indicated that the Corporal had parasite infestations that were causing a disturbance in the large intestine meridian. This was the cause of his undiagnosed abdominal pain. This young soldier could not believe he could have parasites and kept returning to the clinic—to ask me repeatedly, in disbelief, if it was true. I gave him parasite medications with instructions on how to take them (the Army's pharmacy has a very limited selection of parasite medications in the formulary). The soldier did not return for a follow-up visit, and I assume he returned to duty in Iraq.

Meanwhile, I had an opportunity to give lectures on alternative medicine at the U.S. Military hospital. Immediately I received referrals for the most difficult cases in Europe.

One of my last patients that I treated during my deployment was a 49-year-old Colonel. He was a military intelligence officer and a Ranger who served with Special Forces. Colonel H. had a complicated medical and trauma history. He was shot down twice in special operations. Parachute jumps caused multiple breaks in his spine. He was also exposed to depleted uranium and suffered with chronic pain, insomnia, and hypertension for many years. It was amazing to see a man, who had survived multiple physical traumas, still alive and functioning at his level.

The Colonel's first request was to keep him alive so that he could see his 10-year-old daughter get married some day. He knew there was something very wrong with him. Most physicians did not have a full grasp of what was going on in his body.

My Acupuncture Meridian Assessment indicated that he had two main problems: parasites and a hidden dental infection. I gave him parasite medications and told him that, if there was a 50 percent improvement, he could consider that a success. My tour of duty was ending, so I was returning to the U.S.

A few months later, Colonel H. tracked me down. He e-mailed me and explained that his pain was reduced, he was sleeping better, and his blood pressure had responded. Several hypertensive medications that he had previously tried had not been able to control his blood pressure. He had contacted me because his pain and blood pressure were coming back after completing the parasite medication. He was interested in continuing the parasite medication and was seeking a complete recovery.

I asked Colonel H. to write a list of the improvement in his symptoms after taking the parasite medications. I used his testimonial to try to convince four Army medical officers in Germany to give him the same parasite medications, but without success. Nobody has experience using parasite medications. The doctors are afraid to prescribe this type of medication—especially without proof of a lab analysis.

To make a long story short, Colonel H. had great difficulty obtaining the medication he needed. It should not be this difficult to treat our soldiers. Many soldiers are getting less than optimum medical treatment.

I am very proud to have served as a U.S. Army Reserve Medical Officer. I'm also very proud of our capability to treat wounded soldiers with the most advanced trauma care that includes dedicated surgical teams. However, our ability to diagnose and treat complex medical problems is far from ideal. This is obvious from Colonel H.'s story that appears as a patient success story in this book.

I am now retired from the U.S. Army Reserves after 25 years of service. I wonder how I could make an impact on the future medical care of our soldiers. Teaching young medical officers alternative medicine might be the answer, but I'm not sure the U.S. Army is ready for it. At least, not yet. Saving Special Forces Colonel H. made serving in the U.S. Army Reserves worthwhile for me.

Our tour of duty was short, but it has had profound ripple effects on my patients from all over the country. Skeptical patients have become new believers when their "incurable" conditions disappear, thanks to the U.S. Army and my Bolivia Connection.

Fighting Parasite Invaders

If you have read this far in the chapter, or, if you are presently a patient, you are probably wondering:

- If parasites are the cause of most diseases, how does an average person know if he/she has been infected?
- If infected, is a prescription medication necessary to kill a parasite?
- Once a parasite is killed, what preventive measures can be used to avoid reinfection?

The rest of this chapter will address these three questions.

How Do I Know If I Have a Parasite Infection?

People with chronic, unexplained illnesses are most likely infected with a parasite. As I mentioned previously, lab tests for parasites are inadequate. I consider the EAV device to be a valuable tool for identifying parasite infections. One of the reasons that I am writing this book is to inform other physicians about Acupuncture Meridian Assessment. I'm eager to meet medical doctors who would like to learn more about this tool, and I would be happy to share what I've learned.

Is a Prescription Medication Necessary to Kill a Parasite?

In truth, parasites are extremely difficult to kill. When antiparasite medications are used, parasites often move out of the gastrointestinal (GI) tract to avoid the path of a strong drug. When I was in active duty, I was sometimes questioned about prescribing higher-than-normal dosages of antiparasite medications by pharmacy staff who were unfamiliar with parasites.

If you are already a patient of mine and you are reading this, you know that there are many complex issues in the body that make a person vulnerable to disease. A few of these were mentioned at the beginning of the last chapter and listed here as a review:

- Hidden dental infections caused by root canal procedures or an infected cavitation from an improperly extracted tooth (usually a wisdom tooth)

- A decline in the immune system due to inadequate nutrition

- A taxed immune system that is overwhelmed by:

  - Immune-destroying chemicals in food and water

  - Heavy metals

  - Bacteria and other microorganisms in food and water

- Blockages in the body's biocybernetic matrix that lead to signaling errors and altered tissue states

And, as I mentioned in my story about Bolivia, there are several other factors including:

- Food allergies

- Environmental toxicity

- Toxicity in the body

Because vulnerability to disease (and parasite infection) is multi-factorial, there is no silver bullet (or medication) that can eradicate an invader and simultaneously make the body strong enough to resist reinfection. If you have an invader in your body, you will need to

---

The Art of War by Sun Tzu

The *Art of War* is a 2,000-year-old text written by a warrior-philosopher named Sun Tzu. It is recognized as China's oldest military treatise that is well known for its Taoist dimensions. The text, written and preserved on bamboo shoots, presents a philosophy of war that teaches how to win without fighting and how to accomplish the most by doing the least. The *Art of War*, which has gained popularity among military theorists and political leaders all over the world, contains important themes for thwarting an enemy (including parasites—an embedded internal enemy).

---

look at the health of your entire system and build up your body's own defenses to help with the attack and to prevent the invader from getting a foothold in the future.

I have spent the last 15 years developing strategies to assess the presence of heavy metals, identify food allergies, investigate the health of the body's terrain, uncover hidden dental infections, and track the presence of invaders using Acupuncture Meridian Assessment.

If you absolutely cannot see me as a patient, I have added self-help strategies to this chapter that may be tried. These same strategies have also been added for my patients who have killed their parasites with a prescription medication and need a proactive strategy to prevent reinfection.

Understanding Your Strengths and a Parasite's Weaknesses

In the *Art of War*, Sun Tzu suggests an incremental approach to success using small, focused engagements where you have a clear advantage. SunTzu's goal is consistently "victory without battle" or following the easiest path available.

Whether you are in the dark about a possible parasite infection or whether you have already killed parasites with a prescription drug, here are some important concepts and related strategies to remember as you plan your siege:

Directions for Assessing Your Stomach Acid

There are numerous reasons why people may have insufficient stomach acid. Factors may include age, genetics, or low supplies of zinc and protein that are needed to make hydrochloric acid.

A simple test with baking soda can be used to determine if you are producing enough hydrochloric acid. The following steps will reveal whether your hydrochloric acid level is low:

1. First thing in the morning before eating or drinking anything, mix one quarter teaspoon of baking soda in eight ounces of cold water.
2. Drink the baking soda solution.
3. Time how long it takes to belch, and time for up to 5 minutes.
4. If you are producing adequate amounts of hydrochloric acid, you will belch within 2 to 3 minutes. Early and repeated belching is associated with excessive stomach acid. It results from the acid and baking soda reacting to form carbon dioxide gas.

Native American Antiparasite Herbs

Taken together as a single treatment, black walnut hulls, wormwood, and cloves kill the adult and developmental stages of 100 different parasites:

Herb	Source	Target Parasite
Black walnut hull tincture	Black walnut tree	Adult and young worms
Wormwood	Artemisia shrub	Adult and young worms
Cloves	Clove tree	Eggs

It is important to kill all stages of the parasite's development at once because targeting one of the developmental stages will leave others to grow in your body. Dr. Hulda Clark has written several books that contain directions for taking these three herbs as well as sources for purchasing supplies.

Tracking Full and New Moons

The lunar component in parasite reproductive cycles may have something to do with the fact that the Moon causes many of the tides and the fact that life originated in the ocean:

> *At Full Moon and New Moon, the Sun, Earth*
> *and Moon are lined up, producing the higher*
> *than normal tides.*

During a Full Moon and New Moon, parasites detach from the walls of the the body's organs to breed and lay eggs.

Let's explore how you can obtain the information you need to schedule your parasite cleanses around the cycles of the Moon. The following steps will help you create a plan:

1. People who are just beginning a parasite cleanse may need to use antiparasite herbs for several months. Once you have cleared para-

> ### Kroeger Herb Products (www.kroegerherb.com)
>
> Kroeger Herb Products, named after herbalist Hanna Kroeger (1913-1998), is a source for black walnut hull, wormwood, and cloves.

sites, you will need to do a cleanse once or twice a year. Make a decision about the months you plan to do parasite cleanses several months in advance.

2. Purchase a diary to keep track of the months you plan to do your parasite cleanses.

3. Visit the *Farmer's Almanac* Web site to locate the dates for the New and Full Moons in the months you plan to do your cleanses:

   www.almanac.com/astronomy/moon/full/index.php

   Plan your cleanse from a New Moon leading up to a Full Moon and through a Full Moon for several days. *Note: The Moon Phase Calendar available as a link on the Farmer's Almanac Full Moon Calendar page contains helpful graphics for understanding the start of a New Moon and the days leading up to a Full Moon for each month of the year.*

4. Keep a routine going to stay clear of parasites.

Feeding Your White Blood Cells (WBCs)

Hulda Clark's 2007 book titled *The Cure and Prevention of All Cancers* contains helpful information about nutrients that feed the body's white blood cells (WBCs). The following chart contains the nutrients that she suggests as well as food sources:

Nutrient	Food	Notes
Vitamin C	Rose hips	Rose hips contain bioflavonoids rutin and hespiridin that are supporting substances known to increase the effectiveness of Vitamin C.
Selenium	Brazil nuts	Brazil nuts need to be soaked overnight in water with a pinch of salt to loosen phytates present in the outer surface of the nut.
Germanium	Hydrangea root or Korean ginseng	Although Hulda Clark recommends Hydrangea root as a source of germanium, Korean ginseng is very high in germanium, and it is an adaptogenic herb that helps the body to adapt to stresses, such as heat, cold, exertion, trauma, sleep deprivation, toxic exposure, radiation, infection, and psychological stress.

How to Buy Radon-Free Spring Water

If you buy spring water in gallon bottles, select brands that are bottled in high-density polythylene (HDPE) plastic containers that are also filled all the way to the top. When the air space at the top of a bottle is filled, it lowers the risk of radon gas (or polonium, a radon daughter) getting trapped inside.

Situation	Strategy
Path of Entry Although parasites can enter the body through the skin (e.g., through the bottom of the feet), most parasites enter the body in the form of eggs that are hidden in food.	**Assess Your Stomach Acid** Your stomach acid (hydrochloric acid or HCL) kills microscopic parasite eggs that are hidden in food (See: "Directions for Assessing Your Stomach Acid").
Parasites Lay Thousands of Eggs Parasite eggs, larvae, and young worms are easier to kill than adult worms. In 1992, Dr. James H. McKerrow and a team of researchers at the University of California in San Francisco published a report in *Nature* that explained how a species of worms called *Schistosoma mansoni* uses a hormone in the human body called tumor necrosis factor as a stimulant to lay thousands of eggs each day. Schistosomiasis is the disease that is caused by an invasion of this species, and it results from massive reproduction.	**Eradicate Young Parasites** Even though adult worms may be difficult to kill with herbs, botannicals may be used to kill eggs, larvae, and young worms. Examples include: • teas • loose herbs (added to smoothies) Even if you have trouble killing adults, you can halt worm reproduction (See: "Native American Antiparasite Herbs").
Lunar Reproduction Cycles Biological reproduction cycles in nature often have a lunar component that synchronize to a Full or New Moon. This means that parasites come out of their cysts (or hiding places) during a Full or New Moon.	**Follow the Cycles of the Moon** Parasite-killing herbs should be taken a few days before—and through a Full Moon (or New Moon)—to kill newly hatched parasites (See: "Tracking Full and New Moons").

Situation	Strategy
White Blood Cells Need to be Fed White blood cells (WBCs) are an important part of your immune system, and Dr. Hulda Clark has determined what nutrients they need. WBCs are foot soldiers.	**Feed Your WBCs** Take nutrients that feed your body's white blood cells (See: "Feeding Your White Blood Cells").
Worms Contain Bacteria According to Hulda, bacteria can flood the body each time a worm is killed, and bacteria can contain viruses.	**Use Antibacterial Teas** Use teas to kill the bacteria that are released when worms are killed (See: Antibacterial Teas)
Livers Are Destinations for Eggs In an August 1992 *New York Times* article titled, "Worm Uses Hormone of the Immune System to Infect and Multiply" that describes Dr. James H. McKerrow's research at the University of California in San Francisco, McKerrow describes how many eggs (of the *Schistosoma mansoni* worm species) make their way to the liver. He explains, "About half of the eggs burrow through the walls of the intestine or bladder, depending on the species, and are excreted and continue the organism's life cyle. The others are swept into the blood to the liver, where they are encased in granulomas." *Note: There are thousands of worm species that may have similar behavior.*	**Flush Your Liver Four Times a Year** The practice of flushing the liver was used by allopathic medicine in the 1920s and 30s at Boston's Lahey Clinic. The strategy was found by Dr. William Donald Kelley (1925-2005) while he was searching the clinic's archives. Kelley is most known for a protocol that he developed to fight his pancreatic cancer in the 1960s. A liver-gallbladder flush is a proven strategy for removing parasites from liver and gallbladder ducts (See: "Directions for a Liver-Gallbladder Flush").

Antibacterial Teas

The antibacterial teas that Hulda recommends are helpful because worms release bacteria when they are killed. The teas may also be effective in killing young worms in developmental stages. She recommends taking herbal teas for several days in advance of a parasite cleanse to prepare the body for the waves of bacteria that are released. This is a creative strategy that will prevent many symptoms associated with the release of bacteria. Health food stores often sell the loose herbs that Hulda recommends:

- Eucalyptus
- Boneset
- Epazote
- Birch bark
- Burdock
- Reishi mushroom
- Turmeric
- Fennel

Directions for a Gallbladder-Liver Flush

A gallbladder-liver flush is helpful for releasing invaders that have made their home in these organs. It is a quick, easy, and inexpensive way to cleanse the liver, which is considered to be the most important organ system for detoxification.

- **Preliminary Notes**
  - *There are several different recipes for a gallbladder-liver flush. The flush described in this section is based on a recipe that I distribute in my office.*

- *I recommend that a gallbladder-liver flush be done four times a year (similar to an oil change in your car!)*

- *The phosphoric acid that is listed in the recipe should only be used once to help soften gallstones in the gallbladder. This precaution is recommended because phosphoric acid can cause osteoporosis, and it can also harm the enamel on your teeth.*

- *Occasionally, patients need an herbal laxative or several large, warm enemas or colonics to get things moving. If you experience any abdominal discomfort or cramps after the flush, take one additional tablespoon of Epson salt in a 12-ounce glass of water.*

- *A warm water enema or coffee enema can also relieve a Herxheimer reaction if it occurs. A Herxheimer reaction often consists of fever, chills, headache, and muscle pain that is due to a large release of bacteria and toxins. The instructions and supplies for this optional step are provided separately.*

- **Supplies for a Gallbladder-Liver Flush**
    - 1 gallon of organic apple juice (or four quarts)
    - 2 ounces of orthophosphoric acid
      (Phosfood from Standard Process)
    - Epsom salts
    - Extra virgin olive oil
    - Malic acid tablets (100 mg.)
    - Optional beverages for making the olive oil more palatable:

        - Coca Cola and the juice of one whole, fresh lemon
        - Diet Coca Cola for diabetics (this is the only time we recommend Nutra-Sweet)
        - Freshly squeezed pink grapefruit juice (pink grapefruit juice is the most palatable)

- **Supplies for a Warm-Water Enema (Optional)**
  - Enema bag
  - Soft rubber colon tube (See: "Supplies for a Gallbladder-Liver Flush")
  - Spring water

Step #1: Thin Your Bile Three to Four Days Before Your Flush

- Three to four days before you plan to do the flush, pour the entire two-ounce bottle of orthophosphoric acid into the gallon of apple juice. If you have purchased quarts of apple juice, you can add eight full droppers to a quart of apple juice (Note: one full dropper fills about half of the length of the dropper).

- Take one malic acid tablet with each glass of apple juice between meals and drink 3-4 glasses of juice per day. Shake the bottle before you pour the juice. (Option: Rinse your mouth with baking soda or brush your teeth after drinking the juice to prevent the phosphoric acid from damaging the enamel on your teeth.)

- If you have diabetes or a sensitivity to sugar, you may substitute one part apple juice to one part filtered water. Add the eight full droppers of orthophosphoric acid to the diluted apple juice quart mixture.

- Finish the apple juice before you do the flush. Warning: The apple juice and phosphoric acid mixture may cause diarrhea. Do not be alarmed as it will stop on its own.

- Eat light meals.

Step #2: Planning the Evening of the Flush

- On the day of the flush, eat a normal breakfast, lunch, and dinner (Note: Your dinner should be a light, low-fat meal).

- Plan your evening meal so that you can consume 1/2 cup of olive oil at least four hours after your meal.

- Two to three hours prior to drinking the olive oil, mix one teaspoon to one tablespoon of Epsom salt in 12 ounces of water. This Epsom salt mixture is bitter, and you may clear your palate with a lemon wedge. *Note: Epsom salt is optional and is recommended if there is no response to the olive oil.*

Step #3: Drink One-Half Cup of Olive Oil

- After drinking your half cup of olive oil, you will need to lie down for at least a half hour. Because of this requirement, many people plan to take their olive oil at bedtime and just stay in bed for the night.

- Drink 1⁄2 cup of olive oil, mixed with an optional and equal amount of Coca Cola or pink grapefruit juice for taste. Some people add the juice of one whole fresh lemon to the Coca Cola version (this mix should be room temperature).

- Immediately after finishing the olive oil drink, go to bed and lie on the right side with your knees drawn up to your chest for 30 minutes. The olive oil stimulates the liver and gallbladder to purge the contents of your gallbladder and liver. You may feel nausea during the night due to stored toxins that are released from the liver and gallbladder. This is a sign that the procedure is working.

- In the morning, many people will pass hardened gall material that has been nicknamed "greenies." People who have had their gallbladders removed will also see green stones. You will also see cholesterol crystals in the form of small white or tan stones.

- If you do not see any greenies, increase the olive oil to three-quarters of a cup, and then finally to one cup.

Step #4: (Optional) Warm Enema to Rapidly Purge Toxins

- A warm water enema may be used in the middle of the night to relieve nausea or other symptoms that are due to toxins.

- An enema may also be used to get things moving the next day.

- Fill an enema bag with spring water.

- Heat some spring water in a pan and use this warm water to heat the water you have added to your enema bag. The water in the bag should be slightly warm to the touch.

- Find a place to hang your enema bag in your bathroom that is approximately 18-20 inches higher than where you plan to take your enema (e.g., the doorknob if you plan to lie on the floor).

- Insert the colon tube and release the stopper.

   Notes: Releasing the stopper a few seconds before inserting the tube sometimes facilitates an easier insertion. It may be difficult to retain the enema at first.

- Use half of the contents of the enema bag or the entire bag if possible. Try to retain the enema for 10 to 15 minutes.

   Note: You will want to clean your enema bag occasionally with water and liquid soap. Miracle II liquid soap is a a non-toxic liquid soap that is a very effective cleaning agent (See: "Supplies for Gallbladder Liver Flush"). Clamp off the tube and fill the bag with water and half a teaspoon of soap. Rinse your bag thoroughly after 30 minutes.

Research Shows Selenium From Brazil Nuts Is More Bioavailable Than Selenium From Supplements

A study published in the February 2008 issue of the *American Journal of Clinical Nutrition* shows that selenium from brazil nuts is more bioavailable than selenium from selenomethionine supplements.

Researchers from the Department of Human Nutrition at the University of Otago in Dunedin, New Zealand asked a group of adult volunteers to consume either two Brazil nuts (averaging 53 µg. of selenium), 100 µg. of selenium as a supplement, or a placebo for 12 weeks (µg = microgram).

Even though the nuts averaged less selenium, at the end of the 12 weeks:

- The nut eaters had increased their blood levels of selenium by over 64%.

- The supplement takers had increased theirs by 61%.

- The nut eaters had more than twice the blood levels of an important selenium-dependent enzyme, glutathione peroxidise.

The researchers concluded that New Zealanders could avoid the use of supplements and increase their selenium status by including brazil nuts in their diet.

Understanding the Toxins That Get Trapped in Your Liver Ducts

As I mentioned previously, the liver is the most important organ in the body for removing toxic wastes. Under normal circumstances, the gallbladder, the biliary tree (bile's path from the liver to the duodenum), and bile help the liver detox:

- **Bilirubin**
  A brownish-yellow excretion product that is produced when the liver breaks down old red blood cells.

- **Heavy metals**
  Metals with a relatively high atomic mass that can cause damage or death in animals, humans, and plants. Examples include non-organic arsenic, beryllium, cadmium, chromium, lead, manganese, mercury, and nickel.

- **Biotoxins**
  Poisonous substances, especially proteins, that are produced by living cells or organisms.

- **Xenobiotics**
  Drug, pesticides, or carcinogens that are foreign to a living organism.

Patients who have experienced a toxic overload often have toxic deposits in their biliary tree or network of ducts that branch through the liver and gallbladder.

Due to the very high level of pollution in our environment, it is critical that we assist the liver with a flush at intervals throughout the year. Cleaning your liver is as necessary as cleaning your home.

Sources for High-Quality Loose Herbs

The following sources do not disinfect herbs with toxic chemicals:

- Jean's Greens (www.jeansgreens)
- Frontier Natural Products Co-op (www.frontiercoop.com)

Olive Oil Fraud

Author Tom Mueller, who wrote an article called "Slippery Business" for the August 13, 2007 edition of *The New Yorker*, explains that fraud in the international olive oil industry is a major problem.

Fraudulent Practices

Here are some details about the fraudulent practices:

- "Extra Virgin Olive Oil" sold in the United States may be a lesser grade of olive oil or a small amount of olive oil that has been blended with canola or hazelnut oil.

- Olive oil may be derived from olive oil pulp (pomace) left after pressing out the oil. An inferior olive oil can be made from treating pomace with a chemical solvent called hexane.

- The label on an olive oil bottle may contain misleading information about the country of origin. Although most of the olive oil sold in the United States is imported from Italy or Spain, both countries import cheaper oils from Tunisia, Turkey, Morocco, or Libya and use labels that say "Imported from Italy or Spain."

Conclusion

Although a gallbladder liver flush will work with an inferior oil, this chapter offers an opportunity to provide a "heads up" about olive oil fraud. To obtain the health benefits of a monunsaturated olive oil, you will need real olive oil and not a fake substitute. To avoid fraud, you will need to read labels, research a producer on the Internet, and possibly write to the company whose oil you are purchasing.

Gallbladder-Liver Flush: Questions and Answers

I have assembled the following frequently asked questions to help readers learn more about the gallbladder-liver flush.

Question #1: *Do you feel any pain when you do a gallbladder-liver flush?*

> **Answer:** No, however, you may feel nauseated for a few hours. Many people have reported that olive oil mixed with either Coca Cola and lemon juice or freshly squeezed pink grapefruit juice helps to prevent nausea.

Question #2: *Do I have to follow these exact instructions?*

> **Answer:** No, there are many variations of the gallbladder-liver flush. You may do a daily flush with a smaller dose of olive oil, or try different types of oil such as grape seed oil or flax seed oil, if olive oil is not tolerated or available. You may develop your own liver flush recipe (that you will be responsible for).

Question #3: *How long do I have to do this program, and how often?*

> **Answer:** I recommend that you do a gallbladder-liver flush every other week until you pass a few stones, and then monthly. Gradually taper off to four flushes per year (once a season) for maintenance.

Question #4: *If my gallbladder has been removed, can I still do a gallbladder-liver flush?*

> **Answer:** Yes, you will need a flush to get rid of the sludge of bile and toxins in the liver.

Question #5:   *Is there anything dangerous about doing a gallbladder-liver flush?*

Answer: It is possible for gallstones to get stuck in a bile duct and cause acute inflammation of the gallbladder. However, if you use apple juice and the orthophosphoric acid, you should not have any problems (See: "Organic Apple Juice vs. Commercial Apple Juice"). I have never seen a complication as long as you follow all the instructions.

Question #6:   *Are the green objects real stones?*

Answer: The initial bowel passage may contain true gallstones. However, most of the green objects are congealed bile sludge mixed with olive oil that leaves the liver and gallbladder ducts.

Question #7:   *Can I take all my medications while I'm doing a gallbladder-liver flush?*

Answer: Olive oil may upset your stomach, so I recommend that you do not take any medication, vitamins, or minerals for 6 hours before and 6 hours after taking the olive oil.

Question #8:   *Is this the only detox program that I need?*

Answer: Perhaps not. This is a basic, simple detox program. If you are very toxic, you may need a more intense program that includes high enemas or colonics.

Question #9:   *If I don't pass any green objects, should I stop the program?*

Answer: Some people may have to do more than two or three gallbladder-liver flushes before they start seeing green objects. About 60-70% of patients will notice green stones after their first flush.

Supplies for Gallbladder-Liver Flush

- Orthophosphoric acid
  All of the supplies for the liver flush may be purchased at your local health food and drug stores with the exception of the orthophosphoric acid drops. You may order a two-ounce bottle from Ultra Life, Inc.

  Ultra Life, Inc.
  P.O. Box 440
  Carlyle, Illinois 62232
  (618) 594-7711
  Email: ullife@accessus.net
  http://www.ultralifeinc.com

(Optional) Enema Supplies

- Soft Rubber Colon Tube
  Ultra Life also carries a soft rubber tube that can be used with any drugstore enema bag. Attach the long rubber tube to the plastic tip that is supplied with the enema bag.

- Miracle II Soap for Cleaning an Enema Bag
  Miracle II liquid soap is available at the Miracle Merchant Web site:

  www.themiraclemerchant.com

Organic Apple Juice vs. Commercial Apple Juice

The phosphoric acid and malic acid found in apple juice are key ingedients in the gallbladder-liver flush recipe that dissolves and softens gallstones. We have also added malic acid tablets for this purpose.

Some commerical apple juice manufacturers dilute apple juice with less expensive fruit juices, such as white grape juice or pear juice. Natural malic acid is entirely an L-isomer. A pure organic apple juice will have a tart taste that is due to this natural organic acid.

7

Parasites and EAV

*The battle against parasites
is an example of asymmetric warfare*

Asymmetric warfare is a new buzzword that is being used by the American military. Although the word has several meanings, it is often used to describe an enemy that hides in plain site. In the human body, parasites are asymmetric combatants, and there are very few diagnostic tools for today's physicians to identify health problems that are related to these hidden enemies inside the body.

Asymmetric warfare is synonymous with guerilla warfare, a Spanish expression that means "little war." In an asymmetric conflict, the enemy is resourceful and skilled at the element of surprise. Historians who understand innovative asymmetric tactics have identified dozens of examples throughout history, beginning with Hannibal's trip over the Alps that surprised the Romans in 218 B.C. The important distinction that sets the asymmetric enemy apart from a conventional enemy is the ability to hide and adapt rapidly. When a small group of combatants use mobile tactics against a larger enemy, effective countermeasures are needed to:

- **Identify an Invisible Enemy**
  Parasites can move around the body and invade every organ, much like the clandestine guerilla who is a master at cover and

concealment. The Voll machine or electroacupuncture according to Voll (EAV) device is a new biometric tool that can help diagnose a parasite infection. The Voll device monitors the flow of energy to organs via acupoint voltage that is measured on the hands and feet. EAV testing is based on the phenomenon of resonance that has been harnessed in many man-made devices, such as musical instruments, radios, lasers, and medical scanners (e.g. a magnetic resonance imaging [MRI] machine). The EAV device is a meridian-based technology that was developed by a German physician named Dr. Reinhard Voll. Voll's technology uses electrical "norms" or baseline electrical voltages reflecting the energy levels of meridian-associated organs. Through his research, Voll realized that electrical skin resistivity is associated with degenerative disease within an organ system, and high voltage readings are caused by inflammation.

- **Identify a Medication**
  Parasites can be eliminated with herbs, homeopathic remedies, or prescription drugs, and the Voll machine's metal platform provides a means to match the energetic frequency of a parasite

---

Real-Life Medical Tricorders

Star Trek fans have noticed that machines that use energy for diagnostics are not so far-fetched. As of this writing, a handful of real-life tricorder-like devices are cropping up in the United States and Britain.

The original *Star Trek* series, aired in 1966, featured a tricorder that could scan a body and help diagnose and heal injured or sick patients. Forty-one years after Chinese American designer Wah Ming Chang designed the medical tricorder and communicator for Starship Enterprise Chief Medical Officer Leonard McCoy, real-world medical tricorders have finally appeared.

Although the new tricorder-like inventions are very different than the Voll device, all of the machines rely on energy and resonant frequencies for diagnostics.

In November 2007, *Network World* Magazine published an article titled, "Ten Top Real-Life Star Trek Inventions" that includes the University of Washington's Center for Industrial and Medical Ultrasound's tricorder-like tool that doctors can use to scan the body. Writer Michael Cooney noted that Purdue University has also created a hand-held sensor that can be used for testing foods for bacterial contaminants including *Salmonella*. In November 2007, *ZDNet* Healthcare writer Dana Blankenhorn also described an invention created by British Orla Protein Technologies and Japan Radio Co. Ltd. as a "diagnostic biosensor." The hand-held device can perform tests without touching a patient and can transmit the results wirelessly.

infection and and to bring about a remedy. When a medication is placed on the platform, it becomes part of the body's electrical circuit, and the changes that occur in an acupoint reading can help identify a suitable medication.

Parasite Infections Often Go Undiagnosed

If you suffer from unexplained medical problems like chronic fatigue, muscle weakness, fibromyalgia, candidiasis, and anxiety, and your doctor told you every test result is fine, think of chronic parasite infections. Parasite-related problems are one of the most neglected areas of the medical field. Few people recognize that parasites not only cause diarrhea, bloody stools, or abdominal cramps, but also have been associated with a whole list of symptoms, such as anorexia, autoimmune disease, chronic fatigue, constipation, food allergies, gastritis, inflammatory bowel disease, irritable bowel syndrome, low back pain, Crohn's disease, arthritis, headaches, rash, rectal itching, weight loss, and weight gain, and many more.

Parasites Weaken the Immune System

All illness, including parasite infections, develop because one's immune system is weakened. This is indisputable, yet often not acknowledged. Complementary and alternative medicine are based upon this premise. Parasites, which often go undiagnosed, can contribute to a weakened immune system that then allows favorable conditions for a vast range of illnesses to develop. More often, many factors bombard the immune system over time. Parasites are one of several factors that weaken the immune system. Other causes include:

- Heavy-metal toxicity
- Food allergies
- Dental problems
- Poor diet and nutrition

Types of Parasites

In the United States, the most common human parasites are of the microscopic protozoal variety (single cell, amoeba like) that can be transmitted by air, food, water, insects, animals, and other humans. The most common protozoal parasites are *Giardia lamblia, Entamoeba histolytica, Dientamoeba fragilis,* and *Cryptosporidium.* Other types of parasites include pinworms, roundworms, tapeworms, *Trichina spiralis*, hookworms, and *Filaria.*

Dr. Leo Galland, M.D., a New York-based physician who specializes in parasitology, estimates that conservatively a minimum of 10 percent of the American population may be infected by parasites. Worldwide, 25 percent of the population is infected by roundworms, and over 30 percent of the population is infected by protozoal parasites.

The reason that parasites often go undetected is because they do not produce classical diarrheal symptoms or abdominal cramps. Dr. Galland's findings indicate that any person with chronic gastrointestinal complaints,

---

Anne Louise Gittleman's *Guess What Came To Dinner*

In *Guess What Came To Dinner: Parasites and Your Health,* Anne Louise Gittleman says America's parasite problem is a silent epidemic. She explains the dangerous misconception that parasites exist only in tropical areas or among the poor who live in unsanitary conditions. She says the result is a lack of awareness about risk factors and symptoms. Her book provides valuable information on how to prevent parasite infections, including tips about food handling and animal care.

such as bloating, diarrhea, abdominal pain, flatulence, chronic constipation, multiple allergies, and unexplained fatigue, should be screened for parasites.

Stool Specimen Tests Are Unreliable

One of the main reasons that parasites go undiagnosed is because parasitology labs fail to find the majority of intestinal parasites in stool specimens submitted to them. For example, the test of a routine stool evaluation for ova and parasites picks up less than 10 percent of active infections. There are hundreds of parasites with very complicated life cycles that can exist outside the intestinal tract. As a result, they would not be detected by a stool specimen test. Many parasites can penetrate through skin, lungs, nostrils, and every organ and tissue in the body.

The World Health Organization (WHO) has stated that two billion people have worms that are rarely seen in a stool exam. I believe those numbers are very conservative and are limited to worms and nematode infections that do not include all other parasite infections.

Parasite and Allergy Symptoms Compared

I have compiled a chart that lists symptoms associated with parasite infections and allergy-related problems. You will be surprised to see the similarity in the symptoms. Many symptoms that indicate a parasite infestation also indicate allergy problems and vice-versa as shown in the first half of each column. The symptoms in the second half of each column do not mirror each other like the symtoms in the first half, but several of the symptoms seem to influence each other as if running a parallel course.

Parasites	Allergies
Asthma	Asthma
Bloating	Bloating
Brain fog	Brain fog
Cramps	Cramps
Diarrhea	Diarrhea
Fatigue	Fatigue
Flatulence	Flatulence
Gallbladder attack	Gallbladder attack
Headaches	Headaches
Immune deficiency	Immune deficiency
Irritable bowel syndrome	Irritable bowel syndrome
Mucous secretion	Mucous secretion
Muscle problems	Muscle pain
Ulcerative colitis	Ulcerative colitis
Weight gain	Weight gain
Weight loss	Weight loss
Anal itching	Abdominal pain
Appendicitis	Acne
Brain abscess	ADD/ADHD (See: page 73)
Cancer	Anorexia
Cardiomyopathy	Bedwetting
Constipation	Behavioral changes
Cough	Bronchitis
Dermatitis	Canker sores
Eczema	Celiac disease
Fever	Conjunctivitis
General pain	Ear infection
Hallucination	Edema
Indigestion	Hives
Inflammation	Hypoglycemia
Insomnia	Irregular heartbeat
Intestinal bleeding	Irritability
Liver dysfunction	Itching
Malabsorption	Joint pain
Memory loss	Low back pain

Parasites	Allergies
Nausea	Seizures
Peritonitis	Sinusitis
Poor coordination	Skin rash
Pulmonary fibrosis	Urinary problems
Urogenital dysfunction	Urticaria

Treating a Parasite Infection

The treatment plan for parasites included dietary precautions, herbal parasitic remedies, and prescribed medications as indicated. Patients should eliminate all uncooked, raw foods from the diet and cook all meats and fish until well done. Vegetables should be well cleaned, and all sugar should be eliminated from the diet, including fruit juices and honey. Herbal parasite remedies include:

- Citrus seed extract
- *Artemisia annua*
- Wormwood
- Pumpkin seed
- Ginger root
- Black walnut hull extract
- Goldenseal root
- Genitian root
- Clove oil

Patient Success Story
Blocked Breathing From Parasites

At the height of my unexplained physical problems that included back pain, colon problems, uncontrolled facial twitching, panic attacks, and chronic bladder infections, I also had blocked breathing that was frightening. Doctors could not find any physical problems and guessed that I had an atypical, unusual type of asthma.

When I took antiparasite medication, several of my symptoms disappeared—after expelling what looked like a large fluke and pinworms from my mouth and a large tapeworm from my gastrointestinal tract.

For more of this patient's case history and success story,
see page 295.

Notes

8

Food Crimes

*I think that the use of preservatives in food
may be and often is overdone and that great harm
may come from their excessive use.
(From: 1905 Congressional testimony)*

*- Dr. Harvey W. Wiley
Author,
The History of a Crime
Against the Food Law*

This chapter (and the next) contains a collection of food topics that have appeared in my *Healthy Planet* monthly column over the past several years. Food crimes are mostly food myths that have been created by food manufacturers who are interested in selling products.

Food Crime #1: High-Fructose Corn Syrup (HFCS)

Unlike raw sugar from sugar beets or sugar cane, high-fructose corn syrup contains no enzymes, vitamins, or minerals. For people who eat processed foods, such as soft drinks, yogurt, industrial breads, cookies, salad dressing, and soup, this means that the body's reserves of enzymes, vitamins, and minerals are tapped each time these foods are consumed. The result is a dangerous depletion of key minerals that are important to organs such as the heart, elevated blood cholesterol, and a weakening of white blood cells that are important to the immune system. Fructose also reduces the affinity of insulin for its receptor, which leads to Type II diabetes.

Although the Corn Refiners Association would like consumers to believe that high fructose corn syrup is natural, it is really artificially produced using synthetic agents. In HFCS production, corn is milled to produce corn starch, then processed to yield a glucose corn syrup. Later, enzymes, which may be genetically modified, are added to the corn syrup to change the glucose into fructose.

Surprisingly, many health authorities are "sitting on the fence" when it comes to an opinion about high-fructose corn syrup. The Mayo Clinic nutritionist, Katherine Zeratsky, says, "So far, research has yielded conflicting results about the effects of high-fructose corn syrup." Fortunately, the major media has been more decisive. In a news story about the "Sweetener Controversy," published on October 1, 2008, CBS correspondent Kim Lengle revealed that funding for many of the high-fructose corn syrup studies came from companies with a financial stake in the outcome. And, in April, 2009, *New York Times* published Nicholas Bakalar's "Fructose-Sweetened Beverages Linked to Heart Risks" for the paper's Science pages. Quoting a study that was published in *The Journal of Clinical Investigation*, Nicholas wrote:

> *Fructose-sweetened, not glucose-sweetened, beverages increase visceral adiposity and lipids and decrease insulin sensitivity in overweight/obese humans.*

Most Books About Diabetes Do Not Mention High-Fructose Corn Syrup

Surprisingly, most of the currently published books about diabetes do not mention high-fructose corn syrup and a few books *recommend* fructose for diabetics. The authors that recommend fructose for diabetics state that fructose does not cause a rapid rise in blood sugar levels because it must be changed into glucose in the liver to be utilized by the body. Note: The recommendation that diabetics use fructose is old information. See: Other Authors Who Warn Against Fructose.

Enhanced Waters Are Sweetened With HFCS

Enhanced waters such as Glaceau Vitamin Water, Gatorade, and Propel that contain vitamins and antioxidants—also contain high-fructose corn syrup.

Unfortunately, for readers who buy health books, there are only a few authors who are clear about fructose in the form of high-fructose corn syrup. Dr. Julian Whitaker, another well-known alternative medical doctor, is an example. In his *Reversing Diabetes Cookbook*, he says,

We recommend staying away from fructose as a sweetener, especially in the form of high-fructose corn syrup. Even though it has a very low glycemic index and doesn't affect blood sugar much, excessive amounts raise fatty acid and triglyceride levels and interfere with insulin sensitivity. Excesses also contribute to elevated blood pressure and cholesterol that plague many diabetics.

Other Authors Who Warn Against High-Fructose Corn Syrup

Jack Challem, Burton Berkson, M.D., and Melissa Diane Smith, who wrote *Syndrome X*, are another group of contemporary authors who warn readers against the dangers of high-fructose corn syrup. In a section called "The Health Hazards of Fructose," they write:

Many people believe that fructose is a healthy alternative to common table sugar, but there are plenty of reasons to avoid fructose, as well. To begin with, the fructose found in food products today doesn't come from fruit; it's a highly refined product from corn, and there are a number of deleterious health effects attributed to its use.

Food industry forces that support the use of corn syrup are so pervasive that alternative medical doctors often have to refer to studies that were published decades ago to find any references to the negative effects of fructose. For example, Challem, Berkson, and Smith refer to a 1960s physician and researcher named Dr. John Rudkin who noticed that fructose magnified nearly all of the effects found with sucrose. Given Dr. Rudkin's discovery, they say it is ironic that fructose is considered to be a safe sugar for diabetics because it does not trigger a rapid rise in blood sugar. Their report on fructose reinforces what Dr. Wright and Dr. Whitaker have said:

> *Fructose, does, however, do a lot of other things such as increase free-radical production, boost blood levels of cholesterol and triglycerides, and stimulate the production of insulin and cortisol. Also, despite the fact that fructose does not produce a significant increase in glucose level, it does promote insulin resistance. One 1990s study found that the addition of fructose to a fat-containing meal—think of fructose-sweetened cola washing down a cheeseburger—substantially raised post-meal levels of triglycerides.*

[1] Note: The American Diabetes Association (ADA) once recommended fructose to diabetics, but they have since changed their mind. Even though the Corn Refiners Association (www.hfcsfacts.com) continues to refer to positive ADA statements about high-fructose corn syrup on their Web site, the American Diabetes Association's site has links to studies that show the negative consequences of eating high-fructose corn syrup.

In 2005, the ADA entered into a multimillion dollar alliance with Cadbury Schweppes Americas Beverages (CSAB) that may have affected their position on fructose due to the fact that CSAB is the third largest soft drink manufacturer and a manufacturer of candy.

Now that the ADA's 3-year alliance with CSAB has ended, the ADA no longer recommends fructose to diabetics.

USDA Research Shows HFCS Reduces Levels of Calcium and Phosphorus

Challem, Berkson, and Smith also refer to research conducted at the United States Department of Agriculture's (USDA) Agricultural Research Service in Grand Forks, North Dakota. The research shows fructose can increase the likelihood of developing osteoporosis:

Forrest H. Nielsen and David B. Milne placed a group of men on a diet that included five cans of decaffeinated soda (to elimi-nate any caffeine-related effects) sweetened with high-fructose corn syrup each day. The high-fructose soft drinks reduced the men's levels of calcium and phosphorus, which are needed for healthy bones. The effects of fructose were amplified when the men were also placed on a magnesium-deficient diet. Among people consuming refined diets, magnesium intake is marginal because most people do not eat many magnesium-rich foods, such as leafy greens, nuts, and whole grains.

The full text of the Nielsen/Milne study is available on the *Journal of the American College of Nutrition* Web site (www.jacn.org, The interaction between dietary fructose and magnesium adversely affects macromineral homeostasis in men. 2000; (1):31-37).

USDA Economic Research Shows Increased Consumption of HFCS

United States Department of Agriculture research data supports Dr. Jonathan Wright's comments about the increase in consumption of high-fructose corn syrup in the United States (See: chart on the next page). High-fructose corn syrup became an attractive substitute for sugar beginning in 1982 when the United States began putting quotas and tariffs on sugar imports that doubled what the rest of the world pays for sugar. Even though Coca-Cola and Pepsi use sugar to manufacture soft drinks in countries outside the United States, they switched to HFCS in their American-made soft drinks in 1984. The following chart shows that Americans have increased their consumption of HFCS since the early 1980s.

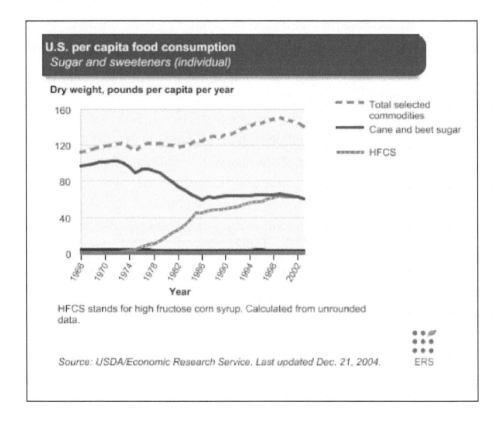

U.S. per capita food consumption
Sugar and sweeteners (individual)

Dry weight, pounds per capita per year

– – – Total selected commodities
——— Cane and beet sugar
▬▬▬ HFCS

Year

HFCS stands for high fructose corn syrup. Calculated from unrounded data.

Source: USDA/Economic Research Service. Last updated Dec. 21, 2004.   ERS

Corn Syrup Was Banned as a Food Additive in 1906!

It is interesting to note that corn syrup was banned as a food additive in 1906 by Dr. Harvey Wiley who is considered to be the Father of the Pure Food and Drugs Act. Wiley was the first head of the Bureau of Chemistry (now the FDA). He banned corn syrup because it was the only sweetener that caused diabetes in all of the bureau's test animals. Ironically, Dr. Wiley predicted that if we ever allowed corn syrup to be used as a food additive, we would become a nation of diabetics. Today, due to pressure from food manufacturers, high-fructose corn syrup seems to be ubiquitous. More than 98 percent of all the food sold in America contains high-fructose corn syrup.

Food Crime #2: Food Additives

Eric Schlosser is an example of a writer who has studied many aspects of the American shift toward processed food and has identified artificial flavors as an important key in the development of processed food manufacturing. In his book, *Fast Food Nation*, Schlosser explains that the food flavor industry emerged in the mid-19th century, as processed foods began to be manufactured on a large scale.

Today, in spite of the popularity of cookbook authors such as Martha Stewart and Rachel Ray, Americans seem too busy to cook. In the 1990s, about 40 percent of all money spent on food away from home went to fast-food restaurants and only 15 percent of the American population regularly cooked at home.

Unfortunately, projections indicate that the percentage of food dollars spent away from home will continue to increase. Estimates place the away-from-home figure at 53 percent in 2010 (up from 27 percent in 1955). If those food dollars are spent on fast food, Americans will be consuming artificial flavors, sweeteners, and preservatives. These *extra* ingredients benefit food manufacturers more than they do our bodies (See: "Ingredients in a Strawberry Milk Shake").

List of Food Additives to Avoid

Today, thousands of chemicals are added to our foods. It is estimated that at least 2,000 of these chemicals have never been tested for potential harmful effects. Private organizations such as the Hyperactive Children Support Group have worked to compile information about the health effects of food additives. Writers such as Dr. Harvey Wiley (See: A Book About Additives That No One Read...), Byron Richards, Randall Fitzgerald, Dr. Earl Mindell, and Dr. Hulda Clark have also helped readers learn about the dangers of chemicals that are routinely added to food (See: Recommended Reading).

The following list of food additives, compiled from several different sources, includes chemicals that have been linked to hyperactivity, attention-deficit disorder (ADD), asthma, cancer, as well as numerous other medical conditions. Note: Because many of the chemicals have alternate names that may not be listed here, it is recommended that you try to avoid food products that contain chemical additives.

H = Hyperactivity

A = Asthma

C = Cancer

Number	Name	Medical Condition		
E102	Tartrazine (food color)	H	A	C
E104	Quinoline Yellow (food color)	H	A	C
E107	Yellow 2G (food color)	H	A	C
E110	Sunset Yellow (Yellow food color #6)	H	A	C
E120	Carmine, Cochineal (food color)	H	A	-
E122	Azorubine, Carmoisine (food color)	H	A	C
E123	Amaranth (Red food color #2)	H	A	C
E124	Ponceau, Brilliant Scarlet (food color)	H	A	C

E127	Erythrosine (Red food color #3)	H	A	C
E128	Red 2G (Red food color)	H	A	C
E129	Allura Red AC (food color)	H	A	C
E131	Patent Blue (food color)	H	A	C
E132	Indigotine, Indigo Carmine (food color)	H	A	C
E133	Brilliant Blue (food color)	H	A	C
E142	Acid Brilliant Green, Green SF, Food Green (food color)	H	A	-
E143	Fast Green (food color)	-	A	-
E150	Caramel (food color)	H	-	-
E151	Brilliant Black (food color)	H	A	C
E154	Brown FK (food color) Food Brown, Kipper Brown	H	A	C
E155	Brown HT (food color) Chocolate Brown HT,	H	A	C
E160b	Annatto Extracts (yellow, red to brown colors)	H	A	-
E173	Aluminium (preservative)	-	-	C
E180	Pigment Rubine Latol Rubine	H	A	C
E200-203	Potassium & Calcium Sorbates, Sorbic Acid (preservatives)	H	A	-
E210	Benzoic Acid (preservatives) Benzene Carboxylic Acid	H	A	C
E211	Sodium Benzoate (preservative)	H	A	-
E212	Potassium Benzoate (preservative)	-	A	-
E213	Calcium Benzoate (preservative)	-	A	-
E214	Methyl Para-hydroxybenzonate (preservative)	-	A	-
E215	Ethyl-p-hydroxybenzoate Sodium Salt (preservative)	-	A	-

E216	Propylparaben Propyl p-hydroxybenzoate (preservative)	-	A	-
E217	Sodium propyl 4-hydroxybenzoate (preservative)	-	A	-
E220	Sulphur Dioxide (preservative) or Sulphur Superoxide	H	A	-
E221	Sodium Sulphite (preservative) or Anhydrous Sodium Sulfite, or Sodium Sulphite	-	A	-
E222	Sodium Hydrogen Sulphite or Sodium Bisulphite (preservative)	-	A	-
E223	Sodium Metabisulphite (preservative) or Pyrosulphurous Acid, Disodium Salt	-	A	-
E224	Potassium Metabisulfite (preservative) or Potassium Pyrosulfite, Pyrosulfurous Acid Dipotassium Salt	-	A	-
E225	Potassium Sulfite (preservative)	-	A	-
E226	Calcium Sulphite (preservative)	-	A	-
E227	Calcium Bisulfite or Calcium Hydrogen Sulphite (preservative)	-	A	-
E228	Potassium Bisulphite, Potassium Hydrogen Sulphite (preservative)	H	A	-
E230	Diphenyl, Biphenyl (preservative)	-	-	C
E231	Orthophenyl Phenol (preservative)	-	-	C
E236	Formic Acid (preservative) or Formylic Acid, Hydrogen Carboxylic Acid, or Methanoic acid	-	-	C
E239	Hexamine, Hexamethylene Tetramine (preservative)	-	-	C
E249	Potassium Nitrate (preservative) or Nitrous Acid Potassium Salt	-	A	C
E250	Sodium Nitrite (preservative)	H	A	C

Ingredients in a Strawberry Milkshake

According to Eric Schlosser, author of *Fast Food Nation*, a typical strawberry milkshake served in a fast food restaurant contains a long list of chemicals. Notice that the list does not contain any milk or strawberries:

> Amyl acetate, amyl butyrate, amyl valerate, anethol, anisyl formate, benzyl acetate, benzyl isobutyrate, butyric acid, cinnamyl isobutyrate, cinnamyl valerate, cognac essential oil, diacetyl, dipropyl ketone, ethyl acetate, ethyl amyl ketone, ethyl butyrate, ethyl cinnamate, ethyl heptanoate, ethyl heptylate, ethyl lactate, ethyl methylphenylglycidate, ethyl nitrate, ethyl propionate, ethyl valerate, heliotropin, hydroxyphenyl-2-butanone (10 percent solution in alcohol), a-ionone, isobutyl anthranilate, isobutyl butyrate, lemon essential oil, maltol, 4-methylacetophenone, methyl anthranilate, methyl benzoate, methyl cinnamate, methyl heptine carbonate, methyl naphthyl ketone, methyl salicylate, mint essential oil, neroli essential oil, nerolin, neryl isobutyrate, orris butter, phenethyl alcohol, rose, rum ether, g-undecalactone, vanillin, and solvent.

Many food companies skip using real food because artificial flavorings are less expensive than real food—reducing the cost for manufacturing. It has become very common to use red coloring instead of strawberries, or orange coloring instead of orange juice, or yellow coloring instead of egg yolks. If you see artificial coloring listed in the ingredients on a package, it is a sign that real food is missing.

E251	Sodium Nitrate (preservative) or Saltpeter, Chile Saltpeter, Cubic Nitre, Nitric Acid Sodium Salt	H	-	C
E252	Potassium Nitrate (preservative)	H	-	C
E260	Acetic Acid, Vinegar (preservative) or, Ethanoic Acid	-	A	-
280 to 283	Propionic Acid (preservative) or Calcium or Potassium or Sodium Propionates	H	A	-
E310	Propyl Gallate (Synthetic Antioxidant)	-	A	C
E311	Octyl Gallate (Synthetic Antioxidant)	-	A	-
E312	Dodecyl Gallate (Synthetic Antioxidant)	-	A	-
E319	Tert-ButylHydroQuinone (TBHQ) (Synthetic Antioxidant)	H	A	-
E320	Butylated Hydroxyanisole (BHA) (Synthetic Antioxidant)	H	A	C
E321	Butylated Hydroxytoluene (BHT) or Butylhydroxytoluene (Synthetic Antioxidant)	H	A	C
E407	Carrageenan (Thickening & Stabilizing Agent)	-	A	C
E413	Tragacanth (Thickener & Emulsifier)	-	A	-
E414	Acacia Gum (Food Stabilizer)	-	A	-
E416	Karaya Gum (Laxative, Food Thickener & Emulsifier)	-	A	-
E421	Mannitol (Artificial Sweetener)	H	-	-
E430	Polyoxyethylene Stearate (Emulsifier)	-	-	C
E431	Polyoxyethylene Stearate (Emulsifier)	-	-	C
E432 - E436	Polyoxyethylene Sorbitan Monolaurate Polyoxyethylene Sorbitan Monooleate Polyoxyethylene Sorbitan Monopalmitate Polyoxyethylene Sorbitan Tristearate	-	-	C
E441	Gelatin (Food Gelling Agent)	-	A	-

Options For Avoiding Dyes in Food

Hulda Clark has discovered that carcinogenic azo dyes "accidentally contaminate" safe dyes such as annatto seed and riboflavin. She tells cancer patients to avoid all dairy products and processed foods.

Rather than buying processed food, an alternative option would be to buy food directly from farmers who do not add chemicals to the food that they sell. Resources for finding farms that sell directly to consumers include:

• LocalHarvest.org
• Weston Price Foundation (network of local chapters, www.westonaprice.org)

E466	Carboxymethylcellulose	-	-	C
E507	Hydrochloric Acid (Hydrolyzing Enhancer & Gelatin Production)	-	-	C
E518	Magnesium Sulphate (Tofu Coagulant)	-	-	C
E536	Potassium Ferrocyanide or Yellow Prussiate of Potash or Potassium Hexacyanoferrate (II) (Anti Caking Agent)	-	A	-
E553 & E553b	Magnesium Silicates Talc (Anticaking, Softener, Agent)	-	-	C
E621	Monosodium Glutamate (MSG), Glutamic Acid, all Glutamates (Flavor Enhancer)	H	A	C
E627	Disodium Guanylate or Sodium 5'-Guanylate, Disodium 5'-Guanylate (Flavor Enhancer)	H	A	-

Code	Description			
E631	Disodium Inosinate 5 (Flavor Enhancers)	-	A	-
E635	Disodium Ribonucleotides 5 (Flavor Enhancer)	-	A	-
E903	Camauba Wax (used in Chewing Gums, Coating and Glazing Agent)	-	-	C
E905 & E905 a,b,c	Paraffin and Vaseline, White Mineral Oil (Solvents, Coating, and Glazing, Antifoaming Agents, Lubricant in Chewing Gums)	-	-	C
E924	Potassium Bromate (Agent used in Bleaching Flour)	-	-	C
E925	Chlorine (Agent used in Bleaching Flour, Bread Enhancer, and Stabilizer)	-	-	C
E926	Chlorine Dioxide (Bleaching Flour and Preservative Agent)	-	-	C
E928	Benzoyl Peroxide (Bleaching Flour and Bread Enhancer)	-	A	-
E950	Potassium Acesulphame (Sweetener)	-	-	C
E951	Aspartame (Sweetener)	H	A	C
E952	Cyclamate and Cyclamic Acid (Sweeteners)	-	-	C
E954	Saccharin (Sweetener)	-	-	C
E1202	Insoluble Polyvinylpyrrolidone (Stabilizer and Clarifying Agent added to Wine, Beer, Pharmaceuticals)	-	-	C
E1403	Bleached Starch (Thickening Agent and Stabilizer)	-	A	-
E1520	Propylene Glycol (solvent for food color)		A	C

A Book About Additives That No One Read...

Dr. Harvey Wiley is often described as the "Father of the U. S. Pure Food and Drug Act of 1906." From 1902 to 1907, Dr. Wiley became the first head of the Bureau of Chemistry that later became the Food and Drug Administration. He was forced from office after 6 years because his work was a threat to food manufacturers.

The title of Wiley's book, which he wrote and self-published in 1929, provides clues about why he left the Bureau of Chemistry:

> *The History of a Crime Against the Food Law: The Amazing Story of the National Food and Drugs Law Intended to Protect the Health of the People, Perverted to Protect Adulteration of Foods and Drugs.*

Harvey died in his home in 1930 and, within weeks after his death, copies of his book disappeared from bookstores and libraries.

Azo Dyes

More than half of all commercial dyes fall within a synthetic category called "azo" that contain a nitrogen "azo group" in their molecular structure. Azo compounds have vivid colors, particularly reds, oranges, and yellows. Azo dyes have been implicated in cancer induction for decades. Due to their carcinogenicity, these dyes have been taken out of the food market, but they are now present in many products in trace amounts.

Notorious Carcinogenic Dyes

Dr. Hulda Clark may be the first contemporary health author to write about "notorious carcinogenic dyes." In her book, *The Cure For All Advanced Cancers*, she says that over 90 percent of the processed foods in U.S. supermarkets is contaminated with unsafe dyes. She identifies the following dyes as the "most notorious carcinogenic dyes:"

- 4-dimethylaminoazobenzene (DAB)
  DAB is the most carcinogenic of the notorious dyes. At one time, DAB was used as a butter colorant and was nicknamed "Butter Yellow." In patients whose blood tests show an elevated alkaline phosphatase, Hulda found an accumulation of DAB in their vital organs and in their fat reservoir.

- Sudan Black B
  Sudan Black B accumulates in any organ, penetrating the nucleus of many cells, making it the most difficult of the dyes to remove. Sudan Black B causes part of the LDH rise that is common in people with advanced cancer. Sudan Black B is found in hair dyes and tatoo chemicals. As a result, only non-carcinogenic natural hair dyes should be used and tatoos should be avoided.

- Fast Green
  Fast Green is not an azo dye but a food color that is used to give fruits and vegetables a more appealing shade. Fast Green contains lanthanide metals—thulium, gadolinium and lanthanum—metals which allow parasite eggs to survive in the body.

- Sudan IV
  Hulda detected a disturbance in the Vitamin A metabolism in organs where Sudan IV (and other azo dyes) are found.

Recommended Reading

The subject of food additives is very large and most of the information is beyond the scope of this book. To learn more about the dangers of food additives, look for the following authors' books:

- Dr. Harvey Wiley, *The History Of a Crime Against the Food Law: The Amazing Story of the National Food and Drugs Law Intended to Protect the Health of the People, Perverted to Protect Adulteration of Foods and Drugs (Note: Philip J. Hilts published a reprint of the original book)*

- Dr. Hulda Clark, *The Cure for All Advanced Cancers (1999), The Prevention of All Cancers (2004), The Cure and Prevention of All Cancers (2007)*

- Russell L. Blaylock, M.D., *Excitoxins: The Taste That Kills*

- Byron J. Richards, *Fight for Your Health: Exposing The FDA's Betrayal of America*

- Kaayla Daniel, *The Whole Soy Story: The Dark Side of America's Favorite Health Food*

Packages that state that annatto seed or riboflavin (natural dyes) have been added, also contain traces of carcinogenic dyes. One of the difficulties is the confusion in the names of the dyes. Sudan IV and DAB have over 40 names each (their popular names are "Scarlet Red" and "Butter Yellow").

Option For Avoiding Dyes in Commercial Hair Color

Hair dye is absorbed by the scalp and remains there in a reservoir to be slowly absorbed for 6 weeks (about the same time that a new batch is applied).

A plant-based dye called henna is safer than hair dyes that contain carcinogenic chemicals. Henna produces a red-orange color, and brown shades are achieved by mixing another plant pigment called indigo.

Mehandi.com is a Web resource for learning how to use body art–quality henna on hair. The company has developed pre-mixed formulas for achieving blonde, brunette, and black shades, and they also provide a free "How-to" e-book about dying hair with henna.

- www.hennaforhair.com (section of the Mehandi site devoted to hair).

Food Crime #3: Cholesterol Therapy Due to Compromised Science

During a patient's first visit, I frequently take them off their cholesterol-lowering medications. Most people who take cholesterol-lowering medication do not understand that the experts who are on the panel for the National Cholesterol Education Program, which sets guidelines for physicians, are on the payroll of the pharmaceutical companies that make cholesterol-lowering drugs (also known as statins).

Quite often, a new patient will say, "My doctor said those medications are for my heart, and I may get a heart attack if I stop." At that point, I have to apologize to my patient and their concerned family members. The truth is, most physicians are not aware of the extent to which medical research has been compromised by commercial arrangements with drug and medical device makers. Aspects of this story have recently been reported in the national press. In a *New York Times* article about Senate scrutiny over the drug industry published on Saturday, July 12, 2008, authors Benedict Carey and Gardiner Harris report:

> *Commercial arrangements are rampant throughout medicine. In the past two decades, drug and device makers have paid tens of thousands of doctors and researchers of all specialties. Worried that this money could taint doctors' research plans or clinical judgment, government agencies, medical journals, and universities have been forced to look more closely at deals' details.*

When it comes to cholesterol-lowering pharmaceuticals, an estimated 13 million people are taking these drugs that have several serious side effects.

Cholesterol Guidelines Have Changed

If you look into the history of "cholesterol guidelines," you'll notice that they suddenly changed 25 years ago, following the now famous Framingham Heart Study. My 1981 laboratory reference book lists a normal cholesterol level for someone who is 50 years old as 150-310 mg/dL. Currently, cholesterol over 200 is considered to be too high for all age groups.

The latest federal guidelines from The National Cholesterol Education Program focuses on lowering low-density lipoprotein (LDL) that is considered to be the main "bad cholesterol." If we follow this guideline, over 40 million Americans will need statin drugs, which represents billions of dollars in sales (a $20 billion market in the United States alone).

Conflicting Stories From Two Framingham Directors

The Framingham Heart Study, now 59 years old, under the direction of the National Heart, Lung, and Blood Institute and in collaboration with Boston University, is one of the largest studies that contradicts the diet-cholesterol-coronary heart disease theory. Although Framingham study director, Dr. William Kannel, made the claim in the early 1980s that total plasma cholesterol is a powerful predictor of death related to coronary heart disease, a decade later in 1992, director Dr. William Castelli, admitted in an article published in the *Archives of Internal Medicine*:

> ... *In Framingham, Massachusetts, the more saturated fat one ate, the more cholesterol one ate, the more calories one ate, the lower the person's serum cholesterol....*

Hypercholesterolemia Is an Invented "Condition"

High cholesterol has been given an official title called "hypercholesterolemia." The term may now be found in the *Merriam-Webster Medical Dictionary*:

> *Presence of excess cholesterol in the blood*

An ad for Lipitor pops up next to the definition in the online version of the *Merriam-Webster Medical Dictionary*.

Dr. Ancel Keys and the Lipid Hypothesis

University of Minnesota professor Ancel Keys first introduced the lipid hypothesis in the 1950s. Although it was his hypothesis that first established a connection between saturated fat, cholesterol in the diet, and the incidence of coronary heart disease, near the end of his life (he died in 2004 at the age of 101), he told an interviewer that, "There's no connection whatsoever between cholesterol in food and cholesterol in the blood. And we've known that all along."

University of Illinois Professor Zeroes in on the Fat Debate

Dr. Clare Hasler, Ph.D., of the University of Illinois, is among a small group of researchers who has had the courage to defend fat as an important component in the human diet. I've mentioned Dr. Hasler's work in this section because there are so few scientists who have taken a stand on the "fat is healthy" side of the cholesterol debate. Interestingly, she zeroes in on the key issue in the debate over fat in a presentation on what are called functional foods. Functional food is an expression that was invented in the late 1990s to refer to a nutritional super-food.

Remarkably, an egg has always been a super-food, but the debate over fats brought a lot of negative publicity that lasted several decades. In a presentation called, "The Changing Face of Functional Foods," Dr. Hasler clears up the confusion when she says eggs have not traditionally been regarded as a functional food, primarily due to concerns about their adverse effects on serum cholesterol levels; she then explains, "…it is now known that there is little, if any, connection between dietary cholesterol and blood cholesterol levels."

Hydrogenated or Trans Fat Causes Heart Disease

In truth, it is hydrogenated fat (or trans fat) that causes heart disease, not animal fat (Note: More information about the connection between hydrogenated fat and heart disease may be found on the Weston A. Price Foundation Web site. An article called "The Oiling of America" provides a very thorough overview of the history and politics of fat (www.westonaprice.org/knowyourfats/oiling.html).

A close look at government health data reveals that myocardial infarction (MI), a blood clot leading to an obstruction of the coronary artery, was almost nonexistent in 1910. Between 1910 and 1990, the total number of deaths per year from coronary heart disease in the United States climbed to almost one million. In this same period, Americans have been told that butter is bad and vegetable oil is good—especially hydrogenated vegetable oil (See: chart).

Understanding Fats

Fats are an extremely complex subject—and many of the details are deliberately left unexplained. The truth is that the companies that make vegetable oil are a powerful force behind the cholesterol myth. The low-fat marketing/public relations campaign originated with the vegetable oil industry (Note: Cholesterol is derived mostly from animal fat and the expression "low fat" or "no fat" is used to promote foods that contain fats derived from vegetables).

Cholesterol is actually good for you. Cholesterol is needed for our cell membranes, our sex hormones, our bile salts, and for our body's production of Vitamin D. We also need cholesterol for proper neurological function and as a protection against cancer and premature aging.

To understand cholesterol, it is helpful to understand the different categories of good fat. *Note: Hydrogenated fat falls into a bad poly-unsaturated category that has been heated to an unnaturally high temperature to prolong shelf life. This processed fat does not fit into the following list of healthy fats that includes two major groups:*

- **Saturated Fat**
  This very important group of fats comprises long chain fatty acids that give cell membranes necessary rigidity. One very essential fact that the fat authorities never mention is that 50 percent of a cell membrane consists of saturated fat. Sources include butter, cream, coconut, palm, cocoa butter, beef tallow, and lard.

- **Unsaturated Fat**
  Unsaturated fats have two major subcategories:

- *Monounsaturated fats*

  This group of fats may be converted to saturated fatty acids (and back) as needed. Monounsaturated fats are known to provide a efficient source of energy.

  Sources include chicken, turkey, goose, and duck fat as well as olives, avocado, and nuts.

- *Polyunsaturated*

  This important group of fats (Omega-3 and Omega-6 fatty acids) react with enzymes to form important derivatives that are critical for our metabolism.

  Sources of Omega-3 fatty acids include fish oil, cold water fish, grass-fed beef, bison, organ meats, and eggs from pastured hens, as well as flax and hemp oil.

  Sources of Omega-6 fatty acids include borage, primrose, black currant, and pumpkin seed oils as well as grass-fed beef and bison, organ meats, and eggs from pastured hens.

Alternative Risk Factors for Cardiovascular Disease

C-reactive protein, homocysteine, and lipoprotein-(a) may give a better prediction for cardiovascular problems than cholesterol. Heavy-metal toxicity and hidden dental infections are also a major source of chronic inflammation and cardiovascular problems.

Food Crime #4: Genetically Modified Organisms (GMOs)

Because polls indicate that 75% of Americans do not know about genetically modified food, I will start this section with a description of a GMO:

A genetically modified organism (GMO) is an organism whose genetic material has been altered using genetic engineering that

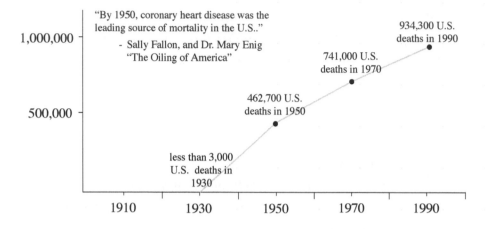

Note: For the last several decades, Americans have been told that butter is bad
and vegetable oil is good—especially hydrogenated vegetable oil (Note:
hydrogenated vegetable oil is another name for trans fat). Source: Sally
Fallon and Dr. Mary Enig, "The Oiling of America."

Multiple Patient Success Stories:
Detoxification With Seed Oils (aka "Oil Pulling")

For reasons that are not scientifically known, high-quality,
cold-pressed, polyunsaturated oil from seeds, such as
pumpkin seeds and sesame seeds, stimulate the body to
detox. I discovered what has become known as an "oil
pull" at a medical conference and later introduced what is
a simple, yet powerful method of detoxing to my patients.
Oil pulling was first introduced by a Russian medical
doctor named Dr. Karach who presented details about the
therapy at a Ukrainian conference of the All Ukranische-
Union of the Oncologists (Specialists for Tumor diseases)

and Bacteriologists (date unknown). To use this powerful therapy, initiate the following steps:

1. Place one tablespoon of sunflower or sesame oil in your mouth when you wake up.

2. Swish the oil around in your mouth for 20 minutes.

3. Spit the oil into the toilet.

4. After the oil has been removed from the mouth, rinse with warm water mixed with half a teaspoon of sea salt and baking soda several times. Brush the gums, teeth, and tongue with the salt and soda mixture.

Notes on oil pulling:

• The oil will be full of toxins and should not be swallowed.

• The oil will change color and appear cloudy when you spit it out.

• If the oil has not changed color, you have not swished it long enough.

• Dr. Karach used this therapy to heal a chronic blood disease of 15 years.

• My patients have solved many complicated medical/dental problems with this therapy.

• Extremely ill patients should do a second oil pull before bed (Also: www.oilpulling.com recommends that an oil pull be done 4 hours after a meal).

is often called recombinant DNA technology. DNA molecules from different sources are combined into one molecule to create a new set of genes (Note: *Escherichia coli* or *E coli* bacteria is a popular organism used in GMO research). The new genes are then transferred into an organism giving it modified traits.

Americans are shielded from news about GMOs because the bio-tech industry has used the services of large public relations firms for crisis management in response to books and videos that have been published by opposition groups. In the last 10 years, PR specialists have told biotech companies to stop publishing research evidence and to refrain from participating in any public debate about GMOs. Due to the very successful news blackout about GMOs, Americans are mostly in the dark about the following:

• Europe and Japan reject GMOs (75% of the world's genetically engineered crops are grown in the U.S. and Argentina).

• More than 90% of the world's genetically engineered seeds have been developed and sold by the Monsanto Corporation (planted predominantly with Monsanto's genetically modified corn, cotton, soybean, and canola seeds).

• Monsanto's genetically engineered (GE) seed sales alone brought the company over $4 billion last year. Outside of GE seeds, Monsanto's past and present product line has included Agent Orange, DDT, PCBs, rBGH, and aspartame.

• A notable historic quote: "Monsanto should not have to vouchsafe the safety of biotech food. Our interest is in selling as much of it as possible. Assuring its safety is the FDA's job." - Phil Angell, Monsanto's director of corporate communications. "Playing God in the Garden," *New York Times Magazine*. October 25, 1998. (See also: "Quotes on the Dangers of Genetically Modified Foods.")

The Dangers Outweigh the Benefits

Recombinant DNA technology first emerged in 1973, and the word "transgenic" is used to describe an organism that has been altered genetically. The biotech industry argues that recombinant DNA technology (also called "horizontal gene transfer") has the following benefits: increased yields, improved resistance to pests, tolerance to herbicides, resistance to disease and drought, as well as a longer shelf life.

One of the world's most respected scientists who has been speaking about the dangers of GMOs is Dr. Mae-Wan Ho, a British citizen from Hong Kong and author of ten books. Speaking at the October 2008 Conference on Future of Food in New Delhi, Dr. Ho provided evidence that is "stacked up against GMOs" in a lecture titled, "Genetically Modified (GM) is Dangerous and Futile." Due to the overwhelming size of the biotech oligopolies, this information is otherwise very hard to obtain. Here is a summary of Dr. Ho's evidence that she presented in her report:

- *No Increase in Yields*
  Studies confirm that the yields of all major genetically modified (GM) crop varieties cultivated are lower than, or at best, equal to yields from non-GM varieties.

- *No Reduction in Pesticides Use*
  USDA data shows that genetically modified (GM) crops increased pesticide use by 50 million pounds from 1996 to 2003 in the United States. (Note: Roundup, a brand name of a systemic, broad-spectrum herbicide used on more than 80 percent of GMO crops planted in the world, is lethal to frogs and toxic to human placental and embryonic cells).

- *GM Crops Harm Wildlife*
  UK's farm scale evaluations and a study led by Loyola University in Chicago have confirmed that GM crops harm wildlife.

- *Forests Have Been Lost to GM Soybeans in Latin America*
  Argentina alone has lost 15 million hectares (Note: One hectare is equal to 2.47 acres). This has worsened considerably with the demand for biofuels.

- *Epidemic of Suicides in the Cotton Belt of India*
  An estimated 100,000 farmers have killed themselves between 1993-2003, and a further 16,000 farmers a year have died since *Bacillus thuringiensis* (Bt) cotton was introduced (Note: Filmmaker Chad Heeter's documentary titled, "Seeds of Suicide" was aired on PBS in July 2005. Heeter's film tells the story of farmers who incurred large debts after being promised greater yields from genetically modified seeds).

- *GM Food and Feed Linked to Death and Sickness*
  Evidence of serious health impacts in lab tests and from farmers' fields around the world.

Note: Dr. Ho's full report is available on the Institute of Science in Society Web site (www.i-sis.org.uk).

Known Risks of GMO Foods

Genetically engineered foods have never been thoroughly studied and scientists are not certain of their safety. Known risks include:

Allergies

If you are allergic to a fish protein that biotech firms are inserting into tomatoes and strawberries to help them with frost resistance, it is very possible that you will be allergic to the tomato or strawberry that contains fish genes.

Antibiotic Resistance

For the past 10 years, numerous cell biologists have been warning about antibiotic resistance caused by GMOs For example, in
a 1998 *Scandinavian University Press* article ("Gene technology
and the gene ecology of infectious diseases." Mae-Won Ho, et al.),
scientists questioned whether genetic engineering that facilitates
what is known as horizontal gene transfer (HGT) is contributing to
outbreaks of drug-resistant diseases.

The Fluid Genome

The technology behind the genetic modification of food is so complex,
it is challenging for the average person to comprehend the consequences
of gene tampering. The dangers of food allergies and antibiotic resistance
exist in a much larger (and much more alarming) context that Dr. Ho
mentions in her recent lecture in New Delhi:

> *...the genome (or the totality of all the DNA in a species) is re-*
> *markably dynamic and "fluid." It is constantly in conversation*
> *with the environment.*

At the beginning of her presentation in New Delhi, Dr. Ho refers to
a headline that appeared in the business section of Britain's *International Herald Tribune* (July 3, 2007) to provide emphasis for her talk:

"Change to Gene Theory Raises New Challenges for Biotech"

According to Dr. Ho, the article went on to say: "The $73.5 billion
global biotech business may soon have to grapple with a discovery that
calls into question the scientific principles on which it was founded."

Dr. Ho went on to explain that genetic engineering of plants and animals
that began in the mid-1970s was based on the belief that the genome is
constant and static. Dr. Ho says that, since the 1970s, a consortium of
researchers who are part of project ENCODE (Encyclopedia of DNA

What Is the Human Genome Project (HGP)?

The Human Genome Project (HGP), a $3 billion project, founded in 1990 by the United States Department of Energy and the U.S. National Institutes of Health, sought to identify the 20,000-25,000 genes of the human body and to study genetic predisposition to diseases.

Elements), organized by the U.S. National Human Genome Research Institute (www.genome.gov/10005107), have discovered that the human body is not made of a "tidy collection of independent genes." Rather, genes "appear to operate in a complex network, and interact and overlap with one another and with other components in ways not yet fully understood." Dr. Ho said that in response to these new findings, The Human Genome Research Institute said this (the ENCODE results) "will challenge scientists to rethink some long-held views about what genes are and what they do."

WARNING: Important Detective Work for People Who Eat in Restaurants: Finding Food That Does Not Contain Sugar

Many national restaurant chains add sugar to nearly all of their dishes (usually in sauces and salad dressings) and baked goods. If you want to successfully manage your insulin secretion, it is important that you inquire whether foods contain sugar. Important factors concerning sugar include:

- Whether you are consuming high-fructose corn syrup that causes diabetes and obesity.

- Whether you are eating sugar from genetically modified sugar beets. Note: American Crystal, a large Minnesota-based sugar company, planned to have (unlabeled) sugar sourced from genetically engineered (GE) sugar beets arrive in stores in 2008. This plan was postponed when the Center for Food Safety (http://truefoodnow.org) won a lawsuit brought against the USDA for approving genetically engineered "Roundup Ready" sugar beets on September 22, 2009. The federal district court for the Northern District of California ruled that the U.S. Department of Agriculture violated the National Environmental Policy Act (NEPA) when it failed to prepare an Environmental Impact Statement before allowing GE sugar beets to be commerically grown. This decision was overruled on March 16, 2010 when a judge in the federal district court for the Northern District of California denied a preliminary injunction to block the use of GE sugar beets. The Center for Food Safety will seek a permanent injunction in July, 2010.

Quotes On the Dangers of Genetically Modified Food

The following quotes are just a *few examples* of notable quotes about GMOs. It is interesting to note that even the Chief Executive of Monsanto admits that the effects of GMOs are unknown.

> *But we realize that with any new and powerful technology with unknown and, to some degree, unknowable effects, there will necessarily be an appropriate level (and maybe even more than that) of public debate and public interest.*

> - Bob Shapiro, October 27, 1998
> Chief Executive of Monsanto
> State of the World Forum (SWF)

Jeffrey M. Smith, who wrote the world's best-selling book about the dangers of GMOs, had this to say about GMOs long before *Britain's International Herald Tribune* 2007's report that there is a change in the gene theory:

> *The current generation of genetically engineered crops is a very primitive technology based on obsolete science that causes massive collateral damage in the DNA that can change proteins and natural compounds in ways that we could never predict. It's an unstable technology, and it was rushed to the market before the science was ready (…). We can link these crops to thousands of sick, sterile, and dead animals, thousands of toxic and allergic reactions in humans, and damage to virtually every system and organ studied in laboratory animals.*

> - Jeffrey Smith
> *Seeds of Deception, 2003*

Jeffrey Smith is also outspoken about the fact that biotech giants rush their patented technology to the marketplace:

> *I asked a scientist who had been fired from his job after 35 years, silenced with threats of a lawsuit, when he discovered that genetically engineered foods caused significant damage to laboratory animals. I asked him what was the most shocking moment. It wasn't being fired from his job; it wasn't discovering the problems. It turned out it was months earlier when he was still a pro-GM scientist in good standing and was asked to review the scientific papers that got GM crops approved in the UK. He said reading those studies was one of the most shocking moments in his life, a turning point in his life, because he realized how bad the research was. He said what they're trying to do is as little as possible to get their foods on the market as quickly as possible. That was his most shocking moment.*

> - Jeffrey Smith
>   *Seeds of Deception*
>   (and *Genetic Roulette, 2007*)

Numerous other scientists from around the world have warned the public about GMOs. Here are just a few examples:

> *Gene technology is driven by bad science. It may well ruin our food supply, destroy biodiversity, and unleash pandemics of antibiotic-resistant infectious diseases.*

> - Dr. Mae-Wan Ho
>   Bio-Electrodynamics Laboratory,
>   Open University in Milton Keynes, UK
>   author, *The Unholy Alliance*, 1997

In an ecosystem, you can always intervene and change something in it, but there's no way of knowing what all the downstream effects will be or how it might affect the environment. We have such a miserably poor understanding of how the organism develops from its DNA that I would be surprised if we don't get one rude shock after another.

> - Professor Richard Lewontin
>   Professor of Genetics, Harvard University

...the allergic potential of these newly introduced microbial proteins is uncertain, unpredictable, and untestable, ...

> - Warning from *The New England Journal of Medicine* in 1996 against the use of microorganisms rather than food plants as gene donors

The genetic modification of food is intrinsically dangerous. It involves making irreversible changes in a random manner to a complex level of life about which little is known. It is inevitable that this hit-and-miss approach will lead to disasters. It must disrupt the natural intelligence of the plant or animal to which it is applied, and lead to health-damaging side effects.

> - *Dr. Geoffrey Clements*
>   *Leader of the Natural Law Party, UK*

9

Food Remedies

He that takes medicine and neglects diet, wastes the skills of the physician.

- Chinese Proverb

In nature, there are foods that have extraordinary powers to rejuvenate, nourish, and cleanse. For years, neighborhood health food stores have been the only source of information about food remedies. Dedicated health food retailers have been a source of books from authors such as Paul Bragg, Jethro Kloss, George Oshawa, Michio Kushi, Bernard Jensen, Ann Wigmore, Adele Davis, Dr. DeForest Jarvis, Dr. Weston Price, Dr. Francis Pottenger, Susun Weed, and Dr. Norman Walker. Through mostly word-of-mouth marketing, these authors have helped keep the tradition of natural, food-based remedies alive. Thankfully, the information has been preserved in spite of the multimillion dollar advertising budgets that help promote processed foods.

Because the subject of food remedies is far too large to fit into one chapter, I have included a recommended reading list and I hope that the food remedies I've selected will prompt readers to search for others.

Remedy #1: Apple Cider Vinegar

I discovered apple cider vinegar in the early stages of my exploration for natural alternative therapies. I was working for an HMO at that time and searching for natural remedies for my patients. I found that apple cider vinegar was particularly helpful for patients with digestive problems. Using apple cider vinegar, my patients were able to stop their antiacid medications. In fact, I tried in vain to convince the pharmacy board members that we could save a lot of money for the HMO by switching from Tagamet and Zantac to apple cider vinegar. When I proposed this at a meeting of medical doctors, as you might guess, I received a cold, silent treatment. Similarly, if you research this subject yourself, you can expect that many health professionals will dismiss the properties of apple cider vinegar as "folksy" and anecdotal. In today's medical circles, anecdotal evidence is considered nonscientific because it is passed along by word of mouth. Ironically, with some remedies, there is a great deal of word-of-mouth evidence, and many remedies have withstood the test of time.

Hippocrates Treated His Patients With Apple Cider Vinegar

Apple cider vinegar was used in the ancient civilizations of Egypt, Babylonia, Greece, and the Roman Empire. It was used for every known medical condition—from simple digestive problems and low endurance to external wound care. In 400 B.C. in Greece, Hippocrates treated his patients with apple cider vinegar and honey for all sorts of ailments.

20th Century Apple Cider Vinegar Gurus

The country's apple cider vinegar gurus (and authors), Paul Bragg and Dr. De Forest Jarvis, lived far away from each other—on the West Coast and the East Coast in the states of California and Vermont:

Paul Bragg (1895 - 1976)

Paul Bragg is perhaps the most famous advocate of apple cider vinegar. His book, *Apple Cider Vinegar, Miracle Health System*, has been sold in health food stores for many decades. Paul was a pioneer in the health field. In 1928, he opened the Health Center of

Los Angeles and wrote a weekly column for the *Los Angeles Times*. Paul's food and publishing company is now run by Patricia Bragg who is a former daughter-in-law.

Dr. DeForest Clinton Jarvis (1881 - 1966)

Dr. DeForest Jarvis' *Folk Medicine*, about Vermont folk remedies, was a best-selling book in the 1960s. Jarvis was an ear, nose, and throat doctor who learned about apple cider vinegar and other remedies from the rural people of Vermont. His book was first published in 1958, it was translated into 12 languages, and sold more than 1 million copies.

Both authors explain that apple cider vinegar is rich in potassium, enzymes, organic acids, minerals, and pectin-soluble fiber. Paul Bragg describes how he watched his father make a drink of water, a teaspoon of honey, and two teaspoons of apple cider vinegar after a long, hard day of farm work. Dr. Jarvis told similar stories about Vermonters using honey and vinegar to recover after hard work— adding that Vermonters "carry heavy daily workloads" and go on well

---

Patricia Bragg's Vinegar Drink

For energy, Patricia Bragg recommends drinking a beverage made with vinegar, honey, and water three times a day (upon arising, midmorning, and midafternoon):

- 1 to 2 teaspoons of Bragg's Vinegar

- 8-ounce glass of water

- 1 to 2 teaspoons of raw honey or organic maple syrup if desired.

This beverage may be made as hot or cold drink.

past "three-score-and-ten years" with good physical and mental vigor, good digestion and eyesight, and good hearing (Note: "three-score-and-ten" is seventy years).

Over 100 Indications for the Medical Use of Apple Cider Vinegar

There are over 100 indications for the medical use of apple cider vinegar and the success of most of the remedies seems to be related to the high potassium content. Examples include:

- Chronic fatigue
- Sore throat
- Mild food poisoning
- Headaches
- Constipation
- Arthritis
- Indigestion
- Dandruff
- Dry skin
- Skin blemishes
- Bladder infection
- Kidney stones

Dr. Alexis Carrel's Chicken Heart

Dr. Alexis Carrel, the first American to receive the Nobel prize in medicine and physiology, and a member of the Rockefeller Institute for Medical Research for 33 years, was an innovative surgeon whose experiments led to advances in the field of surgery and the art of tissue culture. In 1912, Carrel took tissue from the heart of a chicken embryo to demonstrate that cells could be kept alive in the lab. The tissue was kept alive for 34 years through daily monitoring of nutrition, cleansing and elimination. Apple cider vinegar was one of the nutrients given to the cells to

Beware of Fake Apple Cider Vinegar

In the late 1800s, food chemists learned to make acetic acid from coal tar. It is still manufactured today, diluted, and sold as vinegar. By law, the label must say, "diluted acetic acid."

Heinz Apple Cider Vinegar Is Made From Apples

The Heinz apple cider vinegar labels state that it is made from apples. In contrast, Admiration apple cider vinegar does not make this claim. Admiration apple cider vinegar is made by the Supreme Oil Company.

Mother of Vinegar

Raw, unprocessed vinegar bottles contain traces of the microbial mat (the mother) that is responsible for the fermentation. The "mother" can be seen at the bottom of bottled brands such as Paul Bragg's organic apple cider vinegar. The mother of vinegar does not have to be discarded. When you see the mat (or mother) at the bottom of the bottle, you can be assured that the vinegar is real—and contains enzymes and minerals such as potassium, phosphorus, natural sodium, magnesium, sulphur, iron, copper, natural pectin, and trace minerals.

Distilled Vinegar is Good for Cleaning

Imitation vinegar created from diluted acetic acid is a good antiseptic that can be used for cleaning. Due to its low cost, it will always be available on supermarket shelves.

provide a daily quota of potassium. Remarkably, a chicken's life span is about 7 years. The cells outlived Carrel himself—before the experiment was deliberately terminated.

Multiple Patient Success Stories:
Positive Responses From Apple Cider Vinegar

Apple cider vinegar was one of my first introductions to the world of alternative medicine. There were so many positive responses that I observed from simply using one tablespoon of apple cider vinegar with meals, that it was hard not to believe in this natural remedy. It relieves indigestion, bloating, and makes patients simply feel better. To their surprise, many patients were able to stop taking antacid medications.

Patrick, a 57-year-old man who came to see me with a history of chronic indigestion, acid reflux, and bloating is an example of a patient with an apple cider vinegar success story. For many years, Patrick had been taking Zantac for his acid reflux.

Note: The Mayo Clinic defines acid reflux or GERD as a condition in which the liquid content of the stomach backs up into the esophagus causing discomfort and problems with digestion. Alternative medical doctors feel that the problem is too little stomach acid and not too much.

Patrick also had a history of hypertension that was not responding to medication, and he also suffered from general malaise and fatigue. I recommended that he take one tablespoon of Bragg's apple cider vinegar, mixed with 6 to 8 ounces of water, and sip it during his meals. He was skeptical at first and was concerned that the vinegar may exacerbate his acid reflux. To his surprise, not only did his indigestion, acid reflux, and bloating symptoms improve, but his hypertension was also easier to manage, and he noticed more energy.

There are many stories that are similar to Patrick's —
men and women with their own unique story to tell.
Apple cider vinegar is truly a forgotten ancient remedy for
so many chronically ill patients. You can use it for prevention as well as to promote optimal health.

Remedy #2: Raw Food

Raw food is actually man's original diet, often called the caveman's
diet. The earliest humans ate what was available to them in their local environment, which included mostly raw food. For some people,
depending on their metabolic type, raw foods have a phenomenal
rejuvenative power that defies the nutritional programs given by most
conventional and alternative medical professionals. There are several
interesting stories about people who have had miraculous transforma-
tions by eating raw food. A patient of mine named Jeff is an example.

Jeff's Transformation on a Raw Food Diet

Jeff's transformation on a raw food diet helped me understand that
for some people, raw food is very appropriate. He changed my view
of raw food. At one time, Jeff was a muscular 175-pound weight lifter.
Then, rather mysteriously, he became sick and his weight dropped to
80 pounds. He looked old and sickly, and his frail demeanor made
him appear like a concentration camp prisoner. He traveled to major medical centers and health spas, but he could not find a definite
diagnosis or treatment plan. I guided Jeff through an intestinal parasite cleansing, heavy-metal detoxification, and a nutritional program
in my clinic, but Jeff continued to lose weight. In desperation, he
switched to raw foods and consumed the following raw foods:

- Eggs   • Butter
- Meats   • Milk
- Chicken   • Vegetables

Jeff also avoided grains. In a short period of time, Jeff's body made an almost miraculous transformation. At 26, he returned to his previous muscular build.

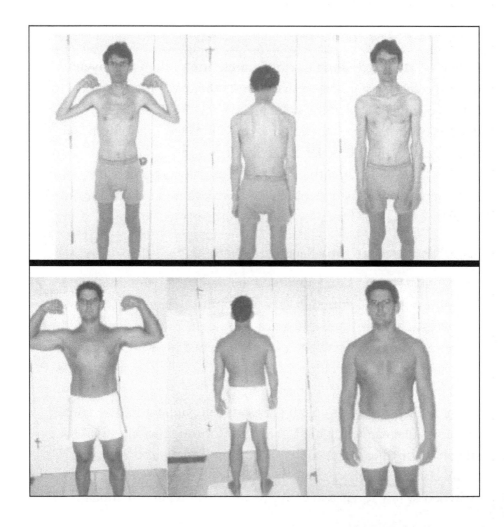

What Is a Raw Food Diet?

By definition, raw food is unprocessed, unheated, uncooked, non-irradiated, nonhomogenized, and unpasteurized. It is typically not genetically modified and frequently organic. Numerous books and nutritional studies have been published throughout the 20th century that explain the reasons why a raw food diet is beneficial:

- *Digestive Enzymes*
  All raw foods contain digestive enzymes (amylases, proteases, and lipases) that aid digestion. These enzymes are destroyed when food is heated above 120 degrees, making it necessary for the body to use its own enzymes to digest food.

- *Beneficial Bacteria*
  Raw foods contain beneficial bacteria and other microorganisms that populate the digestive tract with gut flora.

- *Nutrients Are Destroyed in Cooking*
  In addition to enzymes that are destroyed in cooking, many other nutrients are also destroyed by high temperatures.

- *Cooking Can Produce Toxins*
  Cooking sometimes produces harmful chemicals. Examples include the chemical acrylamide that is a byproduct of cooking starch at high temperatures or glycotoxins that result from heating sugars with proteins or fats.

Dr. Francis Pottenger's Study of Raw Food

One of the most well-known researchers who studied the effect of raw food on nutrition was Dr. Francis Pottenger, Jr. (1901 - 1967). From 1932 to 1942, Pottenger conducted a feeding experiment to determine the effects of heat-processed food on cats.

Prior to his well-known cat study, Pottenger had been conducting a study on adrenal extract and was experiencing a high rate of mortality in the laboratory cats. He noticed that the cats were showing signs of nutritional deficiency, even though he was feeding them raw milk, cod liver oil, and cooked food. All of the cats showed a decrease in their reproductive capacity, and the kittens born in the laboratory had skeletal deformities and organ malfunctions.

Due to his problems with cat health in his adrenal extract studies, Pottenger tried ordering raw meat scraps for a separated group of laboratory cats. Within a few months, the cats in the raw food group gave birth to kittens that were healthier and lived longer. This discovery led Pottenger to undertake a 10-year controlled experiment that helped him to understand the benefits of raw food. His goal was to bring the degenerating cats back to health; he found that it took four generations on raw meat and raw milk to bring the kittens back to normal.

Pottenger's biographers often compare him to Dr. Weston A. Price (1870-1948). Price studied human nutrition in the 1930s and traveled around the world to track the diets of native societies. Over a 10-year period, Price studied the diets of 14 different societies and noticed that human health deteriorated when humans abandoned traditional diets that included many raw foods. Pottenger and Price are obscure names to the general public, but they are highly regarded among alternative health practitioners who study human nutrition.

Contemporary Raw Food Movement

In the 1970s and 80s, raw foods were promoted by health pioneers who helped stimulate the public's interest in nutrition. Examples include authors such as:

Dr. Edward Howell (1898 - 2007)

Dr. Howell was a medical doctor and one of the first researchers to make a connection between enzymes and human nutrition. He is most known for his book, *Enzyme Nutrition.*

Dr. Ann Wigmore (1909 - 1994)

Ann popularized sprouts, wheatgrass juice, and a fermented sprouted-grain drink called rejuvelac. At age 18, after breaking both of her legs in an accident, Ann cured her gangrene with wheatgrass, a remedy that she had learned from her Lithuanian grandmother.

82nd Airborne and Pottenger's Cats: They Don't Make Germans Like They Used To

An article I wrote about my experience at the Army's 325th Field Hospital in Kansas City fits into this chapter.

≈ ≈ ≈

August 1999. In the middle of a hot, muggy summer at Fort Polk, Louisiana, I was doing my U.S. Army Reserve annual training. My home station is the 21st General Hospital in St. Louis, and I was assigned to the 325th Field Hospital in Kansas City. My mission was to support the 82nd Airborne Division for the Joint Readiness Training Center (JRTC) for a joint training exercise with German paratroopers doing night jumps into the swampland at Fort Polk, Louisiana.

Jumping from an airplane with full military gear has a certain rate of injury. Night jump exercises also cause dramatic increases in the injury rate. Our assignment for the 325th Field Hospital was to take care of injured soldiers for the 82nd Airborne Division and the German paratroopers.

We were told to expect greater than a 30 percent injury rate for the paratroopers. We were to be prepared for common injuries from ankle sprains, knee, and back injuries, and occasional dislocations of shoulders and lower extremities. The U.S. Army Reserve medical doctors, nurses, and all the support groups came from all over the Midwest to support the 325th Field Hospital and the 82nd Airborne Division for this joint training exercise.

Every reservist was excited. This was a real field exercise for actual casualties and not our typical mock exercises. Some physicians brought their own medical supplies to treat soldiers. We were ready for the night.

Several hours after the joint exercise commenced, streams of soldiers started coming through the triage area. They were filling the emergency room tent and overflowing to all the medical tents.

I noticed that the wounded 82nd Airborne soldiers and the German paratroopers were on separate sides of the tent. They wore different uniforms, and it was easy to identify them.

Colonel O., an old orthopedic surgeon with a distinct German name, entered the emergency room. He started asking me why there were so many young German paratroopers lined up with injuries. He didn't seem too upset for the 82nd Airborne soldiers lined up with injuries, but was visibly upset and fuming about seeing all those German paratroopers.

I will never forget what he said. "They don't make Germans like they used to!" Almost 10 years later, after

25 years in the Army Reserve, I have retired as a Colonel. However, my memory of that night and his remark are as fresh today as it was at that time. What did he mean?

Without a national or ethnic bias, I think the old Colonel must have been trying to understand the new generation of soldiers. The new generation of young soldiers were not too keen about the old Colonel's attitude of "take the pain, don't complain, learn to live with it."

Attitude does make a difference in how we cope with stress and pain. Since World War II, there's been a gradual change in our attitude toward coping with stress and pain. There has also been a dramatic change in our diet and nutrition. There have been several generations of people who grew up with chemically based, industrial-farmed food. They've been eating highly processed junk foods, laced with chemical additives, for the last several generations.

After all, we *are* what we eat and assimilate. Those modern processed foods often provide maximum calories and minimum required nutrients. They don't provide optimal nutritional support for the body to heal and repair.

In all military branches—the Army, Navy, and Air Force—soldiers are struggling with weight problems very much like most Americans. The basic training for U.S. Army recruits had to be modified because so many young Americans are overweight, out of shape, and vulnerable to a high injury rate.

Those who are interested in nutrition and its effect on human health can look into the Price-Pottenger

Nutrition Foundation (www.ppnf.org). Specifically, refer to "Pottenger's Cats." This was a study in nutrition by Frances Pottenger, Jr., M.D. Pottenger compared cats raised on cooked foods versus raw food and found that the cats on a cooked food diet had an acceleration of physical degeneration, arthritis, sterility, allergies, and skeletal deformities. These cats also passed the deficiencies on to succeeding generations. Also refer to my short article titled, "Raw Food—More Powerful than Most Medicines" among the articles on my Web site.

The 82nd Airborne soldiers, German paratroopers, and Pottengers cats are not much different in regard to the physically degenerative effects of poor nutrition. Generations of changes in eating habits *do* carry their consequences. Rather than saying, "They don't make Germans like they used to," I may add, "They don't make people like they used to, whether German or American." I'm sure the old Colonel would agree with the newly retired Colonel.

Dr. William Donald Kelley Used Raw Food to Recover From Cancer

Dr. William Donald Kelley (1925 - 2005), an orthodontist from Texas, became a proponent of raw food when he cured himself of pancreatic cancer in the 1960s. During the course of his healing, Kelley also discovered that pancreatic enzymes made his tumors shrink. The self-treatment he developed included raw foods and large doses of pancreatic enzymes, which seemed to digest cancer cells.

Kelley introduced his self-help program to cancer victims, and it is estimated that he helped over 100,000 people.

Biochemical Individuality

The raw food diet that Kelley had used to cure his cancer caused him to reformulate his ideas about nutrition. But Kelley's enthusiasm for raw food disappeared when his wife Suzi developed serious health problems—allergies, acute depression, and energy loss to the point of coma. With experimentation and meticulous research, Kelley found that some patients do better on a diet that includes meat. His research helped him develop classifications for people who have different metabolic types. Kelley's classifications are based on the early work of two scientists who pioneered the study of biochemical individuality:

Dr. Roger J. Williams (1893-1988)
Although Williams' name is not widely known, he is considered to be a pioneer in biochemistry and nutrition. Williams was a professor at the University of Texas at Austin from 1939 to 1986 where he discovered the B vitamin, pantothenic acid, and folic acid. During his career, Williams wrote 21 books and over 300 articles. His book, *Biochemical Individuality,* explains that although there are some general rules of nutrition that apply to everyone, each of us has a unique metabolism. In his study of human anatomy, Williams discovered that there are vast differences in the size and structure of human stomachs. He also noted a wide variation in the composition of digestive juices.

Dr. George Watson
Dr. George Watson, a psychochemical researcher at the University of Southern California from the 1950s to the mid-1980s, found biological oxidation rate to be the basis of metabolic individuality.

Watson described oxidation rate as the speed at which the tissues of the body convert food to energy, involving glycolysis, the Kreb's/citric acid cycle and beta oxidation. In his book, *Nutrition and Your Mind* (1972), Watson says that people mostly fall into two distinct groups:

- *Fast Oxidizers*
  This group does well on a diet that is low in carbohydrates but high in fat, purines, and proteins.

- *Slow Oxidizers*
  This group does well on a diet that is low in fat and proteins, but high in salad vegetables and fruit.

Watson used venous blood pH to classify his patients in the oxidation rate categories. Fast oxidizers produce an acid venous blood pH, and slow oxidizers produce an alkaline venous blood pH. He discovered that foods and nutritional supplements can push blood pH too far from 7.46, which is considered an optimal pH. Watson's book contains interesting case studies of people who recovered from illnesses when they made changes in their diets. His research also included vitamin and mineral formulas for each oxidation type.

Kelley's model of metabolic typing has an interesting connection to Francis Pottenger. In 1944, Pottenger wrote a paper called "Autonomic Physiology" that describes how the two branches of the automonic nervous system control metabolism (See: "The Autonomic Nervous System and Digestion"). Kelley blended Pottenger's and Watson's research to formulate his own model of metabolic types that range from slow-oxidizing, sympathetic-dominant vegetarians to fast-oxidizing, parasympathetic meat-eating carnivores.

The Autonomic Nervous System and Digestion

The link between the autonomic nervous system and digestion has been known since Ivan Petrovich Pavlov (1849-1936) studied the link between the autonomic nervous system and digestive system in dogs.

Branches of the Autonomic Nervous System

Hans Selye, an endocrinologist in the 1930s, was the first to identify autonomic and neuroendocrine responses in laboratory animals. From Selye's work, we know the following about the branches of the autonomic nervous system:

Sympathetic branch
The sympathetic branch of the autonomic nervous system controls the body's response to stress, shutting down the gastrointestinal (GI) tract, slowing the liver, and inhibiting the pancreas, thyroid, and adrenals.

Parasympathetic branch
The parasympathetic branch of the autonomic nervous system has a calming effect that increases digestion and increases saliva, liver function, and absorption.

Autonomic Nervous System Dominance Patterns

Kelley noticed autonomic nervous system dominance patterns that form the basis of his metabolic typing model:

Sympathetic Dominant
Some people are born with sympathetic-dominant systems with weak digestion, livers, pancreases, and GI tracts. Sympathetic dominants also have weak thyroids, adrenals, and ovaries. This group has chronic digestive problems. Psychologically, sympathetic dominants tend to

be energetic, they have broken sleep, and although they have short fuses, they tend to get over anger very quickly.

Parasympathetic Dominant

Some people are born with strong parasympathetic systems, with great digestion, and a highly developed liver. Parasympathetics also tend to have a highly developed pancreas and a strong intestinal tract. While this group rarely has digestive problems, they often have allergies, hay fever, sinus problems, viral infections, leukemias, lymphomas, and melanomas. Psychologically, parasympathetic dominants are low keyed, they are prone to depression, and they sleep a lot.

Nutrients and Dominance Patterns

Nutrients can be used to stimulate sympathetic or parasympathetic dominants when they are too far out of balance. Examples include:

Nutrient	Effect
B vitamins	Calm (or weaken) the sympathetic nervous system and stimulate the parasympathetic system.
Magnesium and potassium (high in an alkaline vegetarian diet)	Calm (or weaken) the sympathetic nervous system and stimulate the parasympathetic system.
Calcium, phosphorus, and zinc (high in a meat diet)	Stimulate the sympathetic and calm (or weaken) the parasympathetic nervous system.

One Size Fits All Does Not Work in Nutrition

Health and science reporters often write about new research that is believed to apply to every person's body. Here's an example from a *Washington Post* article titled, "Food as Medicine?"

Tuesday, April 8, 2008 (HealthDay News) — Caffeine, green tea, and tart cherries may guard against multiple sclerosis, cancer, and cardiovascular troubles, respectively, new research suggests.

As Williams, Watson, Kelley and others have discovered, there is no such thing as an "optimal" one-size-fits all diet. Although the research work from these early pioneers is now obscure in a market that is dominated by large pharmaceuticals, their data helps us to understand how chemicals, including the nutrients in food, can have vastly different effects on a person's metabolism.

Nutrient Content in Food Has Dropped By Fifty Percent

It is important to realize that much of our food is very low in minerals that early nutrition researchers discovered had an effect on our autonomic nervous system. Our environment is also much more polluted.

One Man's Meat Is Another Man's Poison

In his philosophical poem, "De Rerum Natura" (On the Nature of Things), Roman poet and philosopher Titus Lucretius Carus (99 B.C. to 55 B.C.) wrote:

Quod ali cibus est aliis fuat acre venenum (What is food to one person may be bitter poison to others).

In March 2001, *Life Extension* magazine published a cover story titled "Vegetables Without Vitamins" that compared the nutrient values in the U.S. Department of Agriculture's food tables published in 2000 to the food tables published in 1975 and 1963. The magazine discovered that the values published in 2000 were numbers that were half of those published in 1963.

Remedy #3: Salt

Most of us know very little about salt—where it comes from, its composition, or why we need it. The information that has formed an impression is mostly incorrect:

- **Salt Is Bad For You**
  For people who are new to the "salt" debate, the "eat less salt" message emerged from the National Heart, Lung, and Blood Institute (NHLBI), and most medical institutions over three decades ago. One of the most significant missing pieces of information in their message is the type of salt. The highly processed bleached form has an unnatural balance of minerals as well as dangerous anti-caking agents.

  The "eat less salt" message is usually accompanied with a warning that salt causes high blood pressure. In an article titled "The (Political) Science of Salt," published in the August 1998 edition of *Science* magazine, American science writer Gary Taubes does an impressive job of separating facts from opinion and brings readers up to date with recent studies that show low-salt diets actually *increase* mortality.

  Interestingly, Dr. John H. Laragh, M.D., at the Hypertension Center of the New York-Cornell Medical Center, says that high blood pressure has nothing to do with salt intake. Overactive hormone systems that produce high renin levels elevate blood pressure. Less than one third of hypertensive patients benefit from a low-salt diet.

- **Iodized Salt is Good For You**
  In the 1920s, public health departments promoted the use of iodized salt to eliminate goiter that is associated with iodine deficiency. A goiter is a noncancerous enlargement of the thyroid gland, visible as a swelling at the front of the neck, that is often associated with an iodine deficiency (usually due to low levels of iodine in the soil). Iodine is required to produce the thyroid hormone, thyroxine, and swelling occurs when the thyroid gland tries to make up for a thyroxine deficiency by increasing in size. Goiters are also associated with inland areas where iodine is very low.

  In the early 1900s, goiter was very prevalent in the states around the Great Lakes, and this area was nicknamed the goiter belt. Other goiter belts include parts of New York, New Hampshire, the Blue Ridge Mountains of West Virginia, and Edmonton, Canada.

  Although visible thyroid problems have disappeared in the United States, there is other evidence of low iodine in this country and other countries of the world:

- **Iodized Salt Provides an Inadequate Amount of Iodine**
  As Dr. David Brownstein points out in his book, *Iodine: Why You Need It, Why You Can't Live Without It*, there is sufficient iodine in iodized salt to prevent goiter, but not enough to prevent thyroid illness or to provide for the body's iodine need.

  Brownstein explains that studies by the National Health and Nutrition Examination Survey I (NHANES, 1971 to 1974) and NHANES 2000 show that urinary iodine levels have dropped

50% in the United States. He says that this drop has been seen in all demographic categories across the United States and that the percentage of pregnant women with low iodine concentration increased 690% in this time period. He further explains that low concentrations of iodine in pregnant women have been shown to increase the risk for cretinism, mental retardation, and possibly attention deficit disorder and other health issues in children.

I recommend iodine for almost all of my patients, espcecially for all women with thyroid conditions, fibrocystic breast, and hormone-related problems. There are many forms of iodine including Lugol's solution. My favorite form is Iodoral tablets that contain iodine and potassium iodide. The tablets are easy to take and widely available.

Understanding How Few Minerals Are in Commercial Salt

Grain and Salt Society founder Jacques de Langre helps readers understand how few minerals there are in commercial salt by comparing it to natural sea salt. In his book, *Sea Salt's Hidden Powers*, de Langre explains that commercial salt has been processed to contain 99% sodium chloride (NaCl) as well as chemical additives to make it bright white and free flowing. In contrast, sea salt contains the following minerals:

Mineral	Percentage in Sea Salt
Sodium & chlorine	84%
Sulphur, magnesium, calcium, potassium	14%
Carbon, bromine, silicon, nitrogen, ammonium, fluorine, phosphorus, iodine, boron, lithium,	1.9997%

Mineral (continued)	Percentage in Sea Salt (continued)
argon, rubidium, copper, barium, helium, indium, molybdenum, nickel, asenic, uranium, manganese, vanadium, aluminum, cobalt, antimony, silver, zinc, krypton, chromium, mercury, neon, cadmium, erbium, germanium, xenon, scandium, gallium, zirconium, lead, bismuth, niobium, thulium, thallium, lanthanum, gold, neodymium, thorium, cerium, cesium, terbium, ytterbium, yttrium, dysprosium, selenium, lutetium, hafnium, gadolinium, praseodymium, tin, berylium, samarium, holmium, tantalum, europium	

Granted, the quantity of these trace minerals in sea salt seems small, but on the other hand, we are talking about nutrients that feed tiny cells. In his book, *Sea Energy Agriculture*, Maynard Murray, M.D., explains that the ocean contains a perfect balance of essential elements that are required as food for the complex cells that make up our bodies. Murray was a medical doctor who researched the importance of trace minerals to plants, animals, and humans. In the 1940s and 50s, Murray used sea solids as fertilizer on vegetables, fruits, and grains. Although Murray has been largely ignored, his experiments demonstrate conclusively that plants fertilized with sea solids and animals fed sea-solid–fertilized feed grow stronger and more resistant to disease. When speaking to farmers about his research, Murray would say, "Life is electrical. Each cell is a little battery that puts out current. Deprived of this function because of nutrient shortfall or imbalance, the cell dies and deprives living tissue of its service."

Most People Are Mineral Depleted

It used to be that you could simply eat a healthy diet to get all the minerals you needed. Today's research shows that this is no longer the case. The nutrient content of our food is on the decline. Soil is the prime source of minerals, and minerals are disappearing from agricultural soils at an alarming rate.

Dr. Linus Pauling, a twice-honored Nobel prize winner, said, "You can trace every sickness, every disease, and every ailment to a mineral deficiency." To obtain the minerals you need, here are a few options:

- Eat organic food
- Use sea salt (1/4 to 1/2 teaspoon to your food)
- Add sea vegetables to your diet
- Take supplements
- Grow your own vegetables (garden soil is probably less depleted than agricultural soils)

Iodoral Tablets From Optimox Corporation

Iodoral tablets, manufactured by Dr. Guy E. Abraham's Optimox Corporation, are a tablet equivalent of Lugol's solution, a formula that is 178 years old (www.optimox.com).

Beware of Bleached Sea Salt

Some vendors sell what they claim to be sea salt, but they are really selling salt that has had all the minerals extracted for other uses. These salt crystals usually look very white compared to sea salt that has an off-white color. Look for the following brands that have had no "anticaking" agents added:

- **Premier Pink Salt**
  This salt is a blend of two unheated, untreated, solar-dried sea salts:

  - Mediterranean sea salt

  - Pink Alaea Hawaiian sea salt mixed with pink Alaea Clay that is rich in minerals.

- **Celtic Sea Salt**
  This hand-harvested salt from *The Grain & Salt Society* is sold in many health food stores and originates from a pristine coastal region in France.

- **EdenFoods Celtic Salt**
  This hand-harvested salt is also from a protected coastal area in France. Eden Foods is a family-owned certified organic producer of over 250 organic products, and their salt is less expensive than the original Celtic Sea Salt.

- **Redmond "Real Salt"**
  Redmond "Real Salt" is mined from ancient sea beds in Utah and not processed with chemicals, additives, or heat. Real Salt has approximately 60 trace minerals, instead of 88 that are available in Celtic Sea Salt.

How Much Salt Is Required Each Day?

Iranian author Dr. F. Batmanghelidj, who wrote *Your Body's Many Cries for Water,* calls a salt-free diet "utterly stupid." He says that in their order of importance, oxygen, water, salt, and potassium rank as the primary elements for survival of the human body.

Although most of Dr. Batmanghelidj's book is about the body's need for water, he explains that we can lose salt from the body when water intake is increased, but salt intake is not. He writes:

> After a few days of taking six or eight or ten glasses of water a day, you should begin to think of adding some salt to your diet. If you begin to feel muscle cramps at night, remember you are becoming salt deficient. Cramps in unexercised muscles most often means a salt shortage in the body. Also, dizziness and feeling faint might be indicators of salt and water shortages in the body.

Dr. Batmanghelidj developed the following rule of thumb for daily salt intake:

> For every 10 glasses of water (about two quarts) one should add a half of teaspoon of salt per day (about three grams).

Accidental Cure for Cancer: A Tribute to Dr. Hulda Clark

As this book was being prepared for publishing, I received news that Dr. Hulda Clark passed away peacefully in her sleep on September 3, 2009 at the age of 81. Many people will miss her as a friend and researcher who made tremendous contributions to our understanding of parasites as a cause of disease. At the time of this writing, a Web site is being set up in memory of Dr. Clark (www. inmemoryofdrhuldaclark.com).

Because most parasites enter the body through food, my article, which is a tribute to Dr. Clark, fits into this chapter on food remedies.

ᴣᴀ ᴣᴀ ᴣᴀ

One of my patients with breast cancer, Janet, gave me a book to read. I read the book. It was written by Hulda Clark, Ph.D., N.D. It was her latest and last book, *The Cure and Prevention of All Cancers*. I was familiar with her work for several years, since I had read her previous books and met her.

In September 2009, I attended the 37th Annual Cancer Convention in Los Angeles, California. At the conference, they announced that Hulda Clark had passed away. I met her on two occasions at another medical conference. She was one of the most brilliant medical research scientists on cancer. She was also a very humble person who had the audacity to write two books with bold claims in their titles, *The Cure For All Diseases* and *The Cure For All Cancer*.

Hulda's theory on cancer is definitely unorthodox, somewhat confusing, and hard to grasp. I won't discuss her latest book that describes every step of how we acquire cancer and how to beat it. I encourage you to read it yourself.

I share many common approaches to cancer with Hulda Clark: parasites, hidden dental problems, heavy metals, allergies, inflammation, nutritional support, and body detoxification. She also explores many topics that seem too esoteric and controversial to understand, given the current thinking in medical science. These need to be further validated. The question is: how muuch validation does conventional medicine need to take her ideas seriously?

Some of my patients beat the odds of dying from cancer despite advanced stages of cancer. Some of them refused surgery, chemotherapy, and radiation. Some went through these same treatments while I was supporting them with nutritional therapy and detoxification. Here are some of their stories:

Florence, an 86-year-old woman from Chicago, came to see me in 1998 with squamous cell cancer of the tongue that had been resected one year before. Note: A resection is the removal of a mass of tissue. Her cancer came back and her doctors wanted her to go through radiation and possibly more resection. Part of my recommendation was to have a biological dentist remove all of her amalgams.

Two months later, I saw Florence, and she told me that her cancer of the tongue had spontaneously resolved one month after half of her amalgams were removed. Her oral surgeon stated he had never observed a spontaneous healing in his medical career. Florence passed away of natural causes at age 94.

Janet, the one who gave me Hulda Clark's book, had a history of breast cancer since 1997. She refused chemotherapy and radiation and came to see me in June 2002. She had three root canals and seven amalgams. During the course of detoxification and nutritional support, she didn't complete her dental work. Her cancer gradually progressed and metastasized to her spine, leg, and pelvic bone.

Later, Janet did finally complete her dental work by extracting the root canals and replacing the amalgams after some initial resistance. She also had multiple rounds of parasite medications, intense detoxification, and intravenous (IV) nutritional therapy with high doses of Vitamin C. Her battle with breast cancer is not yet over, however. She still works part time as a hairdresser, doesn't take any pain medication, and still manages to travel. At the time of this writing (September 2009), she is in Germany visiting her husband's family.

Roseann, an 86-year-old woman, came to see me with a grim prognosis of kidney cancer that had metastasized to her lung. She was told that she had 3 months to live and possibly a slightly longer life expectancy with chemotherapy. She refused chemotherapy and came to see me in August 2007. As part of the treatment, she received parasite medications, Alinia, Praziquantel, and Ivermectin, along with nutritional support and body detoxification programs. As of July 2009, there are no signs of active cancer. She is feeling well and ready to move into a senior apartment for independent living.

Kevin, a 45-year-old man, came to see me in September 2005 with a rare cancer called thymoma (cancer of the thymus) that had metastasized to his lung. He also had myasthenia gravis (muscle weakness). I started him on intense IV nutritional therapy and body detoxification while he was undergoing multiple chemotherapy treatments at the hospital— including experimental chemotherapy medications. He has been one of the few patients who responded to experimental chemotherapy without any obvious side effects.

Is Kevin lucky that conventional therapies are working, or did the additional nutritional therapies and detoxification make a difference? Were all the above-mentioned cases just random luck? Or, is there a legitimately valid methodology in deriving health and healing from this very different perspective compared to conventional medicine's perspective?

My therapy does not target or kill cancer cells. My therapy is designed to support your immune system through a systematic approach to eliminating known toxins, allergens, and infections in the body. Toxins like heavy metals, dental infections, and parasites are eliminated while the patient is provided full nutritional support, including IV nutritional infusions. Some of my patient don't tell their oncologist that they are on nutritional and body detoxification programs. One of the most common comments that I hear from my patients is that their oncologist states that they are "star" patients who respond to chemotherapy, showing minimum signs of side effects.

I believe cancer can be cured with or without chemotherapy, radiation, or surgery, depending on your belief.

I do not treat cancer. I treat the whole body to support the immune system. During this process, you will sometimes observe a spontaneous healing. I call this an "accidental cure for cancer."

This article is a dedication and a tribute to the memory of Dr. Hulda Clark, a brilliant medical scientist, humanitarian, and a humble person with a great concern for humanity.

Notes

10

Peak Performance Diet

*Let your food be your medicine and
your medicine be your food*

*- Hippocrates
460 - 359 B.C.*

merica has the highest obesity rate in the world with 64 percent of adults being overweight or obese. In 2007, the number of obese American adults was estimated at 26.6 percent. Note: The Obesity in America Web site (www.obesityinamerica.org) provides a downloadable file for determining body mass index (BMI), the most common measure of a person's weight, relative to his/her height (See: What Is Obesity?).

Official Dietary Advice Has Failed

After three decades of advice about a low-fat diet, we can conclude that this approach has failed. To understand the relationship between diet and fat, you don't need to seek the advice of a nutrition specialist. Just ask a pig farmer and he/she will tell you:

If you want to fatten pigs, feed them grains and corn. If you want lean meat, feed them a high-fat diet.

The World Health Organization estimates that between 1995 and 2000, the obese population worldwide increased by 100 million (to 300 million). The response to this news has been surprising. Instead

What Is Obesity?

Many Americans who are obese do not understand that they are excessively overweight. So, who decides who is fat and who is obese? The World Health Organization defines obesity as a very high amount of body fat in relation to:

- Lean body mass
- Body mass index (BMI) of 30 or higher

The body mass index (BMI) is a measurement system that became popular in the 1950s and 60s. World Health Organization guidelines set the normal/overweight cut-off at a BMI of 25.

History of Body Mass Index

The body mass index (BMI) formula was created by Belgian statistician Adolphe Quelet (1796-1874). BMI is also referred to as "body mass indicator." To calculate his index, Quelet used the following formula:

$$BMI = \frac{\text{Weight in pounds}}{(\text{Height in inches})^2} \times 703$$

Do the Math to Face the Truth About Your Weight

The Body Mass Index formula works for about 75 percent of the population. It does not work well for children or athletes (See: The Problem With the BMI Formula). To face the truth about your weight, it helps to work out the math and look at a chart that lists the international categories for underweight, normal, overweight, and obese.

1. Take your height in inches and square the number (multiply the number of inches by the same number of inches).

2. Divide your weight in pounds by your height in inches squared.

3. Multiply that answer by 703. The answer is your Body Mass Index.

Weight Categories
Different nations of the world use different BMI ranges to classify weight status. The following table is in keeping with the internationally recognized U.S. Department of Health & Human Services weight status categories.

BMI	Weight Category
Below 18.5	Underweight
18.5 - 24.9	Normal
25 - 29.9	Overweight
30 & Above	Obese

The Problem With the BMI Formula
Although Quelet's formula works for most people, gender and age variables are not taken into account. In addition, BMI does not work for highly toned athletes. Because muscle tends to be heavy, athletes often have a high BMI, even though they are not overweight or obese. These discrepancies were solved in early 1990s when a Japanese company called Tanita introduced a scanner that has settings for children and athletes (See: "Bioelectrical Impedance Analysis [BIA]" on the next page).

Bioelectrical Impedance Analysis (BIA)

Because body mass index data does not work for every-one, I use an electronic body composition monitor called Innerscan to provide patients with in-depth information about several variables that affect their health including:

- Weight
- Body fat percentage
- Body water percentage
- Daily caloric intake, or estimated number of calories that can be consumed within the next 24 hours in order to maintain a patient's current weight
- Metabolic age rating that compares basal metabolic rate to the average age associated with that level of metabolism
- Visceral fat, or the fat in the abdominal cavity surrounding vital organs
- Muscle mass, the weight of muscle in a patient's body
- Bone mass or the weight of bone in a patient's body

Tanita, an electronic scale manufacturer in Japan, introduced the world's first Innerscan body composition analyzer/scale to doctors in 1992 and developed the first home monitor in 1994. The device uses electrical impedance, or opposition to the flow of an electric current through body tissues to calculate body com-position. Child, adult, and athlete modes compensate for discrep-ancies that occur when using the BMI formula.

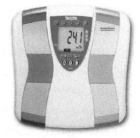

Home Monitor

of finding ways to encourage people to lose weight, businesses are creating things that are "plus size." A few examples include:

- **A Resort Built for Obese People**
  In Cancun, Mexico, a resort called Freedom Paradise has billed itself as the world's first resort designed for obese people by providing amenities such as large armless chairs, wide steps with railings in swimming pools, walk-in showers instead of bathtubs, and stronger hammocks.

- **An Online Retailer That Sells Large Products**
  An online retailer called Amplestuff.com is selling seatbelt extenders, large umbrellas, large clothing hangers, large towels, and scales that can accommodate up to 1,000 pounds.

Chronic Disease Statistics Have Increased

Chronic diseases are long-term illnesses, such as heart disease, asthma, cancer and diabetes. They are the leading causes of death and disability in the United States:

- 133 million or 45% of the population have at least one chronic disease.

- Chronic diseases are responsible for 7 out of every 10 deaths in the United States, killing more than 1.7 million people in the United States every year.

A Poor Diet Weakens the Immune System

Illness develops because one's immune system is weakened. This is indisputable, yet often not acknowledged. Complementary and alternative medicine is based on this premise. Although illness is often related to many factors that bombard the immune system over time, an important factor is poor nutrition.

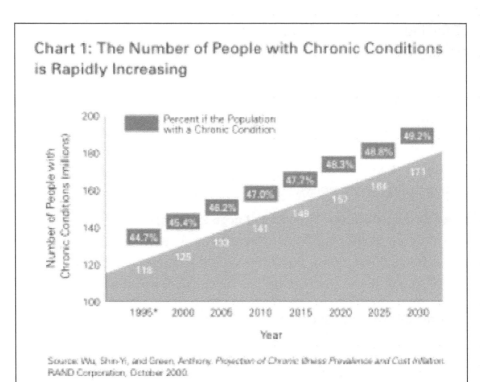

Chart 1: The Number of People with Chronic Conditions is Rapidly Increasing

Dr. Barry Sears' Zone Diet Provides Peak Performance

Author Barry Sears, Ph.D., whose *Enter the Zone* was published in 1995, says his concept of *The Zone* was strongly ridiculed when he first came up with the idea in the 1980s. Now that he has written eight *Zone* books, and the *Zone* is on the verge of becoming what he calls a "mainstream nutritional program," he explains that some of his "most vociferous past critics are now adopting many of the *Zone* concepts as their own." Here is some interesting background information about the *Zone*:

- *The Zone* is an expression that Sears uses to describe a state of feeling energized, happy, and satisfied. In contrast, if you're "not in the Zone," you feel exhausted, hungry, and down in the dumps.

- The media has incorrectly referred to *The Zone* diet as a high-protein diet. As Barry Sears explains, it is not a high-anything diet, but a diet that balances protein, carbohydrate, and fat at every meal.

- *The Zone* diet was originally developed for treating cardiovascular disease and Type 2 diabetes.

- Sears' father died in 1972 at the age of 54. After watching every male on his father's side die as a result of premature heart attacks, Sears was determined to take care of his personal health status by changing his own eating habits.

- After 20 years of research, he learned that food can indirectly turn genes on and off by altering the levels of hormones in our bodies.

- The underlying goal of *The Zone* is to control hormones. Sears' books teach readers to treat food with the same respect as any prescription drug and calls insulin one of the most powerful hormones in our body.

- In many ways, *The Zone* is about keeping insulin levels within a "zone"—not too high and not too low.

  It's food that regulates our insulin levels. Food is really more powerful than medicine for your overall health.

- Barry has invented a clever hand-eye method for calculating portion size that frees his readers from the need to calculate calories. This concept is very well defined in the *Zone* Primer chapter in his latest book called *The Top 100 Zone Foods*.

Barry Sears' Dinner Plate

For meal preparation and portion control, a dinner plate illustrates how to balance portions of protein, carbohydrate, and fat at every meal.

Fill the protein section with a portion no bigger than the size and thickness of your palm and fill the other two-thirds with carbohydrates from *The Zone's* high-quality fruit and vegetable list (Note: Snacks may be assembled in a similar way on a dessert plate):

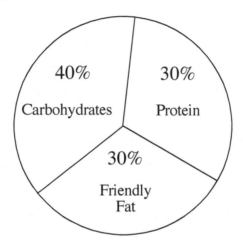

Eat five times a day:

- Three *Zone* meals

- Two *Zone* snacks

Eating five times a day is just one of the *Zone* Rules that also includes the following basics:

1. Always eat a *Zone* meal within one hour after waking.

2. Every time you eat, go for a *Zone* balance of protein, carbohydrate, and fat.

3. Snacks or *Zone* mini-meals are consumed in the late afternoon and late evening.

4. Never let more than five hours go by without eating a *Zone* meal — even if you're not hungry.

5. Eat more fruits and vegetables and ease off bread, pasta, grains, and other starches.

6. Drink at least 3 to 4 8-ounce glasses of water each day.

7. If you make a mistake at a meal, don't worry. Mistakes made at meals can be made up at a subsequent meal—to move your hormones back into the *Zone*.

Carbohydrates Are the Reason You Are Fat

Barry Sears and Dr. Robert Atkins wrote the first diet books teaching a basic diet principle that pig farmers already knew:

*Carbohydrates are the
reason you're fat.*

Although the Sears' and Atkins' diets are somewhat different, they both stand out among numerous other diet book authors who tell people to eat a low-fat, high-carbohydrate diet. That advice has had a devastating effect. The dietary advice that was supposed to help people lose weight actually made them gain a lot of weight.

Understanding the Difference Between Sears and Atkins

Robert Atkins (1930 - 2003) promoted a low-carbohydrate diet that emphasizes protein and fat intake in addition to leafy vegetables and dietary supplements. Barry Sears promotes a middle-of-the-road diet that limits carbohydrates in a 40-30-30 plan or 40% carbohydrates, 30% protein, and 30% fat.

Of these two low-carbohydrate diets, the Atkins diet is higher in fat and is suited for patients who are fast oxidizers. Oxidation rate refers to the conversion of food to energy; people who oxidize food quickly need heavier proteins and fat as emphasized on the Atkins diet. Slow oxidizers do much better on Sears' Zone diet.

In my practice, I have discovered that about 10 to 15 percent of my patients are fast oxidizers. Most people are slow oxidizers and would feel uncomfortable on a diet of slow-burning foods. Because they burn food more slowly than fast oxidizers, they need a complement of fast- and slow-burning foods.

Barry Sears' Breakthrough

While the dietary establishment was telling people to eat carbohydrates (they still do), Barry had the good sense to ask:

*What happens when you
eat too much carbohydrates?*

The storage capacity for carbohydrates in the human body is limited:

- 300-400 grams in your muscles (inaccessible)
- 60-90 grams in your liver

Once these levels are filled, excess carbohydrates are converted to fat. The excess carbs also cause an excessive secretion of insulin, a storage hormone that can cause several other negative effects in the body including:

- Increased blood pressure
- Elevated cholesterol
- Fluid retention
- Arterial damage
- Accelerated aging

Understanding How Insulin Can Push Your Body Out of the Zone

When you consume carbohydrates or sugar, the body produces glucose that is sent into the bloodstream. When this occurs, the body reacts by secreting insulin. The more carbohydrates that you consume at a meal, the more insulin is secreted.

Insulin activates or inhibits many metabolic pathways that can make a person feel sleepy, hungry, dizzy, stuporous (dazed or foggy), or bloated. Barry Sears would consider all of these states to be "out of the Zone."

There are no drugs available to significantly reduce insulin levels. Dietary management is the only effective treatment for excess insulin and the side effects of hyperinsulinemia (See: What Is Hyperinsulinemia?).

Case Study: Patient Lost 30 Pounds and Reduced Insulin When He Cut Carbs From His Diet

Although most of my patient case studies are in Part 4 (Patient Success Stories and Testimonials), this short case study, containing my clinical notes about a Type II diabetic, fits into this chapter.

Chief Complaint: A 64-year-old man with a history of brittle Type II diabetes came to see me in January 2007.

Note: The term "brittle" is used when a person's blood sugar level frequently swings (and swings quickly) from high to low and from low to high. Brittle diabetes is also called labile and unstable diabetes.

The patient was overweight (258 lbs/ 5'8" with 35% body fat mass) and also had a history of hypertension, coronary artery disease with a history of heart attack, and stent placement in 1999. He was also on 160 units of insulin per day for his brittle diabetes.

Treatment: After diagnostics and a physical exam, the patient started intestinal cleansing and parasite medication (tinadazole), based on the results of an Acupuncture Meridian Assessment. Other treatments that were introduced to produce beneficial effects included:

- A low-carbohydrate diet with a nutritional regimen that was based on a hair mineral analysis and a food allergy test.

- Instructions to stop all insulin but to add metformin and to use insulin as needed, based on a finger-prick test for blood sugar.

- Intravenous (IV) EDTA chelation therapy for multiple heavy metal exposure.

Results: The patient was able to lose 30 pounds, and his blood-sugar level became stable without using insulin.

Searching for Food Allergies to Fine-Tune the *Zone* Diet

In my practice, I have watched patients lose weight, feel better, and gain energy on the *Zone* diet. However, I have also noticed that some people do not respond as favorably. For these people, the culprits may be food allergies and a blood-type incompatibility that may be triggered by proteins in food (See: More Fine-Tuning With a Blood-Type Diet).

The incidence of food allergy is much higher than what is documented (See: The Emerging Allergen-Free Market). Food allergy not only causes a variety of cutaneous (skin), gastrointestinal, and respiratory problems, but it also contributes to chronic fatigue, headaches, depression, sinus infections, palpitations, fluid retention, behavioral

---

What Is Hyperinsulinemia?

Hyperinsulinemia is a condition in which there is too much insulin circulating in the blood. While a patient who has hyperinsulinemia may not be diabetic, the condition is often present in Type II diabetics.

---

problems, as well as disturbances of the central nervous system. The most common, everyday foods in the American diet that have been shown to induce allergic reactions include:

- Wheat
- Dairy products
- Corn
- Eggs
- Citrus products
- Soy
- Peanuts

Alternative Doctors and Delayed-Onset Food Allergies

Conventional medical doctors believe that classic or immediate-onset food allergies are the only real allergies. Because the incidence of food allergies is increasing, it is helpful to understand the difference between classic food allergies (IgE mediated) and delayed-onset (IgG mediated). The distinction will help you have an important conversation with your doctor:

- **Classic Food Allergies**
  This type of food allergy is also called immediate onset, and it occurs in 2 to 5 percent of the population. This form is common

in children and rare in adults. IgE mediated means that the body's immune system creates an antibody called immunoglobulin E (IgE) to certain foods. When a person with this type of food allergy eats an allergic food, chemicals are released by large blood cells called mast cells, causing a reaction in various target organs. Reactions may include skin eruptions, respiratory reactions, headaches, gastrointestinal symptoms, and possibly a life-threatening reaction called an anaphylactic response. Anaphylaxis occurs in several target organs at once and is usually very rapid.

- **Delayed-Onset Allergies**
  Delayed-onset allergies involve a different antibody called immunoglobulin G (IgG). Because conventional and alternative medicine disagree over whether this form of food allergy exists, this type of allergy is often referred to as a food intolerance. IgG antibodies do not involve mast cells but bind to food allergens as they enter the bloodstream. Delayed-onset refers to the fact that the symptoms can appear anywhere from a couple of hours to several days after consuming an offending food. This form of food allergy is considered to be elusive because there are several hundred different symptoms that may be triggered.

In my practice, I routinely order blood tests that screen for IgG food allergies. The report that is produced from these tests is invaluable because it alerts the patient to offending foods that need to be eliminated from the diet. Important notes: Offending foods can often be added back into the diet when a patient's antibodies have calmed down. This usually takes anywhere from 6 months to 1 year. Although food avoidance is the primary treatment option for foods that appear in a "highly allergic" category on a food allergy test report, I have discovered a few homeopathic remedies that counteract food allergy symptoms.

The IgG food allergy report that I receive is color coded to flag allergic foods. A highly allergic food is coded with a +3, a moderately allergic reaction is coded with a +2, and a food with a low allergic reaction is coded with a +1. In the black-and-white chart below, I have circled scores on a patient's chart that indicate the most important foods to be eliminated (+3 and +2).

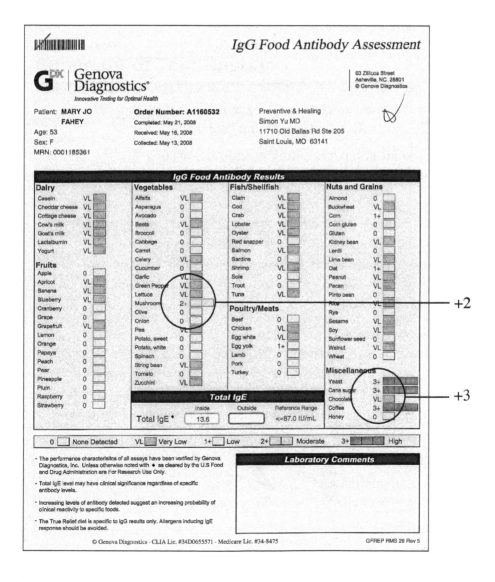

Peanut: A Poor Man's #1 Super Food That Is Packed With Nutrition (After Raw Eggs)

Peanuts, a legume first cultivated by the Incan Indians in 2,500 B.C., are so dense with nutrition, they may be considered a "super food." Besides potassium and monounsaturated fat, which both provide energy, peanuts other benefits include:

- High in protein (27%, needed for tissue repair)

- A source of dietary fiber

- 13 Vitamins (including A, B group, C, and E) and 26 minerals including calcium and iron

- The fat in peanut butter is used for making hormones and vitamin D

Note: In 1921, scientist George Washington Carver (one of America's most famous black scientists) was given 10 minutes to speak to Congress about the peanut—on behalf of the Peanut Growers Association. Members of Congress were so fascinated with his talk, he spoke for an hour and a half.

Peanuts Are Subject to Mold

Aflatoxin is a metabolite produced by two species of mold (*Aspergillus flavus* and *Aspergillus parasiticus*) that form on peanuts and several other foods. Contamination depends on agricultural practices and the susceptibility of food to fungus during storage and processing.

Peanut Allergy

As acupuncturist, Heidi Hawkins, explains in an article titled "Mold allergy," written for the April 2004 edition of

Acupuncture Today magazine, peanut allergy is nearly always an allergy to aflatoxin. She explains that this toxin is formed on peanuts, corn, wheat, soy, tree nuts, oil seeds, and sorghum. Aflatoxin is sometimes measured in milk excreted by cows fed moldy feed.

Prevention of the Formation of Aflatoxin

Prevention of the formation of aflatoxin relies on avoidance of contamination after harvest using rapid drying and good storage practices. Lots of contaminated peanuts can be detected and sorted with electronic equipment.

How Prevalent Is Aflatoxin?

In countries that carefully inspect imported food, very low levels of aflatoxin have been reported. In Japan, inspections for aflatoxin in 1999 and 2000 indicated that 6.9% of 5,108 samples were contaminated with aflatoxin at levels ranging from .2 to 760 $\mu g/kg$ (Note: μg or mcg are abbreviations for microgram, which is one millionth of a gram).

Buy High-Quality Peanut Butter

Cheap supermarket peanut butter is much more likely to contain aflatoxin than better brands. Look for high-quality peanut butter in the natural foods sections of supermarkets or health food stores.

More Fine-Tuning with a Blood-Type Diet

In 1996, Dr. Peter J. D'Adamo put a new twist on dietary guidelines when he published *Eat Right For Your Type*, a book that correlates a body's chemical reaction to food proteins with blood type. I have discovered that patients who are not all that successful with the *Zone* diet often find success if they add Dr. D'Adamo's guidelines for blood types that are described in his book. My office provides blood-type lists that organize recommended foods for each of the blood types into the following categories:

- **Highly Beneficial**
  D'Adamo calls this group "foods that act like good medicine."

- **Neutral**
  According to D'Adamo, this group includes "foods that act like foods."

- **Avoid**
  This group causes the most problems and may be considered to be a poison for people who have a blood-type incompatibility.

Although food lists can help you select the correct foods for your type, I highly recommend Dr. D'Adamo's book.

When you follow Dr. Barry Sears' Zone diet, a food-allergy rotation diet, and Dr. Peter D'Adamo's blood-type diet, you will notice a surge of energy and a gradual improvement from all sorts of ailments, such as eczema, hypoglycemia, and arthritic pain. You will also notice that it is easier to shed pounds. Be sure to visit my Web site and see how I have combined these strategies in an article called "Peak Performance Diet."

Dr. D'Adamo's Online Food List

Dr. Peter D'Adamo's Web site contains a Blood-Type Diet/ Nutrient Value Encyclopedia that lists compatibility details for hundreds of foods. See: www.dadamo.com/typebase4/ typeindexer.htm

Part 3

My Articles

Notes

11

Food-Related Articles

*Half of what you eat keeps you alive, the other half keeps
doctors alive (eat —but remember you have
a choice about the half that you eat).*

- *Simon Yu, M.D.*

For over 10 years, I have been writing articles about my medical research and success with therapies that the world refers to as "alternative." Fortunately, St. Louis has a natural living magazine that has provided me with a platform to share my information with the public. *The Healthy Planet* magazine, now in its 13th year, was founded by J.B. Lester and his wife, Niki. As this book was being prepared for publishing, J.B. commented that when he started his magazine, the words alternative and wellness were considered to be "out on the fringe," but today, most conventional health organizations use these two words. J.B. and his wife work to connect health, wellness, and the environment—concepts that they feel cannot be separated. Readers who have read this far in the book know that I agree with these two publishing pioneers.

This chapter, like the two that follow, contains a few of my favorite articles that were originally published in *The Healthy Planet*.

Aspartame, the Sweet Deception

This article was co-authored by a medical student named Aaron and was titled, "Aspartame, the Sweet Deception: A Medical Student's Story on Diet Soda." At the time that we wrote this article, I had the privilege of teaching third-year medical students from Washington University's School of Medicine. Students spent 1 month with me in my private practice. For a student, this is called a preceptorship. Students have an opportunity to observe and learn an integrated approach to medicine that combines internal medicine with alternative medicine.

When I met Aaron, I noticed that he was drinking diet soda. Most diet sodas contain aspartame. I gave him the assignment of investigating the potential dangers of this toxin and asked him to prepare a written report as though he were preparing a lecture for his patients about the dangers of aspartame. The following is Aaron's story on aspartame:

ಶ ಶ ಶ

When I started my month with Dr. Yu, I came into a world of confusion. Dr. Yu revealed to me ideas and a real-world understanding of medicine, based on actual results, which challenged the concepts I had learned in medical school. Many of the ideas were contrary to the paradigms and standards of medicine that had been imprinted into my mind.

The weeks that followed challenged the reality of what I had been taught to be "truth." It was not long before my eyes were opened to the harsh reality of modern medicine driven almost exclusively by the monetary gain of the pharmaceutical companies.

Aspartame, also known as Nutrasweet, Candrelel, or Equal, was a serendipitous discovery in 1965 by James Schlatter, a chemist working for G.D. Searle & Company. In 1981, Arthur Hull Hayes, a Food and Drug Administration (FDA) commissioner, approved aspartame for use in dry goods. In 1983, the FDA further approved aspartame for use in carbonated beverages.

In 1993, the FDA approved aspartame for use in other beverages, baked goods, and confections. In 1996, the FDA removed all restrictions from aspartame, allowing it to be used in all foods. *These approvals came, even in the face of evidence that aspartame may have negative effects on health.*

Since its categorical approval, *aspartame has been blamed for causing up to 92 different symptoms*, including, most commonly, headaches, dizziness, changes in mood, and nausea. While these complaints have been filed with the FDA, no formal investigation (outside of surveys) has taken place. In addition, 10 percent of aspartame by weight is broken down into methanol and formaldehyde, both of which are chemicals known to have adverse effects on the human body.

A study done in 1998 looked at the distribution of radio-labeled aspartame in mice. It found parts of aspartame bound to the DNA and protein in the liver, kidney, and brain. Another part of aspartame, phenylalanine, is a neurotransmitter in the brain. There are speculations as to whether the sudden increase in the blood level of this neurotransmitter causes adverse effects.

Perhaps more disturbing than the above is the controversy over whether aspartame causes cancer. A 7-year study, published in 2005, followed 1800 rats with varying levels of aspartame modeled after human consumption. This study found increased levels of lymphomas, leukemias, peripheral nerve tumors, and kidney cancers.

In addition, there are basic science studies that support the idea that aspartame may cause cancer. In one experiment with mice, aspartame was found to increase levels of cancer genes in the bone marrow and the kidney. These are the same affected body areas as the first study.

Why, then, is there so much controversy over the safety of aspartame? For every study, there are many more studies "disproving" the dangers of aspartame. Indeed, the medical literature seems filled with studies asserting the safety of aspartame. It is no wonder that the medical community seems to have reached a consensus that aspartame is not dangerous.

However, a review of the literature found that 100% of the studies funded by the aspartame industry asserted the safety of aspartame. However, 92 percent of the independently funded studies found adverse reactions with aspartame! This large discrepancy raises great suspicion as to the validity of the industry-funded studies and whether those studies have been tainted by financial incentives.

As medical research is conducted, it is imperative to consider the financial incentives and ties of the researchers. One must also discern the influences and underlying motives behind the driving forces of the industry. The lies surrounding aspartame are a clear example of the "bias" dangers within the current medical system and government approvals.

While medical doctors cannot be excused for their lack of objectivity, I know that as I continue in my medical training, I will not let rose-tinted glasses color my perception of reality. I will educate those around me, doctors and patients alike.

Soybean Heads: Deception and Dark Side of the Soybean Miracle

I wrote this article in spite of the fact that St. Louis is the heart of corn and soybean country (it's Monsanto's corporate headquarters).

るん るん るん

I believe there are millions of people who have been deceived. Unknowingly they have been converted into "soybean heads" who believe in the "soybean miracle." The soybean miracle implies that soy can save humankind from protein starvation, help women with menopausal symptoms, prevent breast and prostate cancer, and is as near a perfect food as can exist.

One cannot dare tell a soybean head not to eat soy without a lecture coming back at you on the infinite virtues of soy. Soybean heads try to convert everyone to soy products of all types. They believe soy should be eaten in all forms. They tell you that if you're not feeling up to par, just eat more soy. The irony is that soy may be the reason you're not up to par in the first place.

I don't blame these individuals. I'm not making fun of them either, just jesting with them. However, I am very serious about their buy-in to a deception. Why am I so concerned about the unrestricted use of soy products?

Soybeans came into common use in China during the Chou dynasty (1134-246 B.C.). The soybean was considered one of the five sacred grains, along with barley, wheat, millet, and rice. However, the soy plant was initially used as animal feed and crop rotation. Soy is a legume, which means it puts nitrogen back into the soil. Therefore, after a field is grown with crops that deplete the nitrogen from the soil, soy would be grown in the field and nitrogen would be added back to the soil.

Soybeans were not used for human consumption until some time during the Chou dynasty. At that time, soybeans were consumed by humans only as the fermented products of tempeh, natto, miso, and soy sauce. Fermented soy is very different than unfermented soy.

Later, the Chinese were able to precipitate soybeans with calcium sulfate or magnesium sulfate to make a smooth bean curd called tofu. Tofu is not a fermented product. Soy then became widely used throughout Asia. Soy products have been traditionally served with other foods like fish broth, sea food, pork, and other meats. Soy was not the major source of protein in Asian diets.

Today, millions of Americans are consuming soy milk and soy formula. Women especially are consuming soy for menopausal symptoms. Many infants are being fed soy formulas. Soy milk and soy infant formula have never existed in human history until now.

We are in a giant human experiment on a grand scale. Some of the symptoms caused by soy include acne, canker sores, inflammation and infection of the mucous membrane lining of the eyelids and conjunctiva, dermatitis, diarrhea, eczema, hives, heart palpitation, irritable bowel syndrome (IBS), panic attacks, and PMS-like symptoms. I conservatively estimate about 10 percent of my patients are allergic to soy. Many of them don't even know this until we test them.

One of the major side effects of soy is that it blocks the absorption of essential minerals. This results from soy's high content of phytic acid or phytates that especially block zinc, calcium, magnesium, and iron. Only a long period of fermentation will significantly reduce the phytate contents of soybeans. Tofu and soy milk have a high content of phytates.

Other negative effects include the following: soy has an estrogenic effect from the isoflavones and goitrogenic (suppressing thyroid function) effects. Soy also contains trypsin inhibitors (growth inhibitor) and hemagglutinin, a blood clot–forming substance. These negative antinutrient and toxic effects of soy cause a far more harmful impact than a beneficial impact.

Soy protein alone does not provide all the essential amino acids. It needs to be supplemented with lysine, either from grains, eggs, dairy, nuts, or spirulina. Textured vegetable protein is created by subjecting soybeans to high temperature, high pressure, and the use of acid and alkaline chemicals. Artificial flavorings are then added to cover up the unpleasant taste. This process does not create a healthy food.

There has been a tragic misunderstanding about soy. Soy products that are not fermented have been regarded in the same light as fermented products. But these are vastly different. Fermented soy products have been thought of as the same industrial, chemically processed textured soy protein products. However, this is not true. Fermented soy has been used for thousands of years in Asia. Fermented soy products reduce or eliminate the phytic acid and phytates in soy.

Although soy protein isolate has been classified with GRAS (generally recognized as safe) status just like casein protein from milk, there is overwhelming evidence to cause great concern regarding soybean products. I am not trying to be an alarmist and add more fear to an already confused public. I think that you must be informed to protect yourself and your family. Soy can be a valuable protein source in limited use. You can enjoy fine Asian foods in the form of miso and tempeh with soy sauce.

However, I strongly urge all patients to avoid unfermented soy products like soy milk and soy yogurt. Consume tofu in moderation for 1-2 servings per week. Dairy products have been demonized for the use of bovine growth hormone in cows. However, given a choice, unless you are allergic to milk protein, cheese is a better option than soy products.

You can get organic cheese and dairy products from cows that are not raised with growth hormones and antibiotics. Also, goat's milk may be a good choice. Goat's milk is easier to digest and less allergenic than cow's milk and has similar protein and calcium content. For more information on soy, you can look at a study done by Mary Enig, Ph.D., at www.ratical.org/ratville/soydangers.html.

Vitamin D: Power of Darkness, Ray of Hope

In this article, I ask the question: *Is there a "power of darkness" promoting deceitful information about the danger of natural sunlight?* With cancer as the number one cause of death and the number of patients with autoimmune diseases steadily rising, it appears that this may be the case.

Since the 1940s, researchers have noticed that there is a higher incidence of hypertension, colon, prostate, and breast cancers among people living in the mid and high latitudes (Note: latitude is the distance north or south of the equator, which is explained at the end of the article). At first, scientists could not explain the connection, but eventually realized that temperate zones get less sunlight, which means the people living there get less Vitamin D.

꙳ ꙳ ꙳

Vitamin D is not a true vitamin. Vitamin D is actually a steroid hormone. Vitamin D hormone deficiency is a worldwide problem. The most well-known Vitamin D deficiencies are rickets and osteomalacia from defective bone development. We need Vitamin D to absorb calcium and build strong bones.

Over the last 10 years, the latest medical science indicates Vitamin D deficiency has also been associated with an increased incidence of cancer, autoimmune diseases such as multiple sclerosis and rheumatoid arthritis, inflammatory bowel disease, and Type I diabetes. It is also associated with hypertension, chronic pain, obesity, influenza (flu), tuberculosis, heart disease, and accelerated aging.

Vitamin D deficiency has been associated with autism. Dr. John Cannell, M.D., the Executive Director of the Vitamin D Council, has written extensively on the subject of autism and describes a child who recovered from autism with a high-dose (5,000 international units/day [IU] Vitamin D) regimen. The child had a mutated Vitamin D receptor.

Most people understand that we need sunlight with ultraviolet radiation (photons) to convert cholesterol in the skin to synthesize

Vitamin D3 (cholecalciferol). Four Ultraviolet B photons combine with one molecule of cholesterol to make Vitamin D3. However, Vitamin D3 is not a biologically active hormone. It is a prehormone. It needs to be converted to 25 hydroxy Vitamin D3 in the liver and finally converted to biologically active 1,25 dihydroxy Vitamin D3 in the kidneys.

For the last 50 years, there have been strong recommendations to avoid sun exposure and increase the use of sun block lotions to prevent skin cancer and damage to the skin. It became medical heresy to recommend sun tanning in any form. During that time period, there has been a dramatic increase in the incidence of every form of chronic illness from cancer to autoimmune diseases, as mentioned above. These are new, modern plagues. *The medical scientific community has been looking at DNA and a genetic basis as the cause of the new modern plagues, but are we missing something as simple as sunlight?*

Niels Ryberg Finsen, who received the 1903 Nobel Prize for Medicine for recognition of his work and treatment of tuberculosis and lupus erythematosis with UV light radiation, opened a new avenue for medical science. With his discovery, sun spas developed in Europe. In 1919, Huldschinsky cured childhood rickets with sunlight.

Is there a "power of darkness" promoting deceitful information about the danger of natural sunlight? Fortunately, there is overwhelming evidence pointing to the sun's UV radiation in moderation as possibly one of the most cost-effective ways to prevent these modern plagues. After all, sunlight is free!

Why does Vitamin D hormone therapy improve so many different medical problems? Among its many roles, Vitamin D modulates DNA at the cellular level. It strengthens the innate immune system by producing antimicrobial peptides (ll-37), also called "cathelicidin," to combat infections and heal wounds. Vitamin D3 induces cathelicidin to kill tubercule bacilli and fight influenza (flu) viral infections.

Why is flu season in the winter time? Why do people feel sad or easily depressed when the weather is cold and gloomy from December through February? You don't need a Ph.D. in science or a medical degree to figure this out. Fifty percent of hospitalized patients are deficient in Vitamin D according to a major medical journal (Holick, *Mayo Clinic Proceedings*, 2006).

I've been measuring Vitamin D by measuring the level of 25-hydroxy Vitamin D3. Most people are very low or low normal on a scale of 20-100 nanograms per mililiter (ng/mL) reference range. The optimal level should be 50-65 ng/mL. For cancer patients, this should be elevated to a range of 65-90 ng/mL. Most people can take 2,000 to 3,000 IU of Vitamin D3 without concern for side effects. It is a good idea to check your level 3 months after starting Vitamin D supplements.

Cancers strongly sensitive to Vitamin D include breast, colon, prostate, lymphoma, bladder, ovarian, endometrial, gallbladder, stomach, pancreatic, kidney, and rectal. Moderate Vitamin D-sensitive cancers include leukemia, lung, melanoma, multiple myeloma, small intestine, vulvar, and thyroid.

The liver and kidneys play very important roles in converting Vitamin D3 to the biologically active 1,25 dihydroxy Vitamin D3. These organs are very susceptible to heavy-metal toxicity and environmental chemical exposure. Total-body detoxification with specific liver and kidney cleansing programs is an imperative step for prevention and healing for whatever ails you.

Get sunlight, but don't get sunburn. We cannot get adequate amounts of Vitamin D from food alone. Most adults need to take at least 2,000 to 3,000 IU of Vitamin D3. If you're under a doctor's supervision, measure your Vitamin D level. Not all Vitamin D is the same. Some Vitamin D is synthetic. Avoid prescribed synthetic Vitamin D given in 50,000 IU pills. It is not a natural Vitamin D3, but a Vitamin D2 called ergocalciferol. *Sunshine is natural, free, and the absence of darkness: our ray of hope.*

Your ability to safely generate Vitamin D from the sun will be determined by the climate where you live and your skin type. The climate where you live is determined by your location and something called latitude that is defined as the distance north or south of the Earth's equator. If you remember from grade school geography class, latitude lines are horizontal and longitude lines are vertical. Because these lines intersect, they help navigators describe any location on earth. The earth's equator divides the globe into a Northern and Southern hemisphere, and the equator has a latitude of zero degrees.

ঽঌ ঽঌ ঽঌ

In his book, *The UV Advantage*, Dr. Michael Holick divides the world into four main climate regions:

- Tropics (0 degrees to 23 degrees)
- Subtropics (23 degrees to 35 degrees)
- Mid latitudes (35 degrees to 50 degrees)
- High latitudes (50 degrees to 70 degrees)

While it's impossible for people in the mid and high latitudes to make Vitamin D in the winter months, Michael Holick says it is possible for some people to safely generate enough Vitamin D from May to October to last through the winter months.

This article draws material from lectures by the following: Coleen Hayes, Ph.D., on "Sunlight, Vitamin D, and Autoimmune Disease,"

Cynthia Browne, M.D., on "The role of Vitamin D in carcinogenesis," Joseph Mercola, D.O., on "How sunshine reduces cancer by fifty percent" and the Vitamin D Council (vitamindcouncil.org).

Apple Cider Vinegar: A Forgotten Ancient Remedy

This article was originally titled, "Apple Cider Vinegar, Forgotten Ancient Remedy: A Holy Grail for the Fountain of Youth."

ð ð ð

"Apple cider vinegar for the fountain of youth? You must be kidding!" you may say. How about those new, exotic fruit drinks from Tibet, China, or the Pacific Islands? On the other hand, what about the old adages like "an apple a day keeps the doctor away?" And what of the old European folk tale that says, "An apple a day keeps the doctor begging for bread?"

Perhaps the apple and apple cider vinegar have hidden powers as elixirs that have been forgotten in search of the allure of newer, exotic fruit drinks from mysterious, remote mountains or islands. Or does our attention simply get quickly diverted with the latest "FDA-approved" magic bullet medications?

On the other hand, the latest statistics, as reported in the *Journal of the American Medical Association* (*JAMA*) in 2001, indicate that prescription drugs and medical therapies are one of the leading causes of death in the United States after heart disease and cancer.

In the early stage of my exploration for natural alternative therapies for my patients, while I was working for an HMO, I had great success using apple cider vinegar with my patients who had all sorts of digestive problems. However, for the last 15 years, even I have forgotten the benefits of using apple cider vinegar.

Using apple cider vinegar, many patients are able to stop antacid medications. In fact, I tried in vain to convince the pharmacy board members that we could save a lot of money for the HMO by switching Tagamet and Zantac to apple cider vinegar. When I proposed this at a meeting of medical doctors, as you might guess, I received a cold, silent treatment. I stopped using it out of humiliation.

Apple cider vinegar was used in the ancient civilizations of Egypt, Babylonia, Greece, and the Roman Empire. It was used for every known medical condition from simple digestive problems, for endurance and stamina, and for external wound care. In 400 B.C., in Greece, Hippocrates treated his patients with apple cider vinegar and honey for all sorts of ailments.

Why is apple cider vinegar such a powerful antiaging elixir? Should it be considered a holy grail of the fountain of youth? Paul Bragg, N.D., Ph.D., described it best. In his book, he describes the virtue of apple cider vinegar: "It helps to promote a youthful skin and a vibrant healthy body, helps remove artery plaque and body toxins, fights germs, bacteria, viruses, and mold naturally, helps regulate the calcium metabolism, helps digestion, assimilation, balances the pH, helps banish aches, athlete's foot, soothes burns, helps fight arthritis, and helps control and normalize body weight."

Apple cider vinegar is rich in potassium, enzymes, and many organic acids. It also contains minerals like boron, iron, trace elements, and pectin-soluble fiber. Potassium is considered the mineral of youthfulness. It helps the arteries stay flexible and resilient, and maintains youthful, healthy skin. Potassium deficiency can stunt growth. A shortened life span occurs for people living on foods that are grown on potassium-deficient soil.

The organic acids like acetic acid, lactic acid, and propionic acid promote digestion, balance acid/alkaline levels of the blood, help detoxify the body, dissolve fats, and kill viruses, bacteria, and fungus.

Dr. Alexis Carrell, Nobel Laureate in medicine in 1912, from the Rockefeller Institute for Medical Research in New York, kept the cells of a chicken heart alive and healthy for over 35 years by daily monitoring their nutrition, cleansing, and elimination. A chicken's full life span is about 7 years. Apple cider vinegar was one of the nutrients given to the chicken heart cells daily for its full quota of potassium.

Carrell stopped the experiment after 35 years of keeping the chicken heart cells alive and stated, "The cell is immortal. It is merely the fluid it floats in that degenerates. Renew this fluid at intervals, give the cells what they require for nutrition and, as far as we know, the pulsation of life may go on forever."

Achieving immortality may not be possible or desirable, but with good nutrition and healthy life styles, we may lead active lives up to 120 years like the Hunzas of Kashmir and the Georgians of Russia.

Well, are you ready to feel younger? Let's start the day with apple cider vinegar! You may start with one teaspoon of apple cider vinegar mixed with eight ounces of filtered water. Gradually increase this to two tablespoons with your meal.

There are well over 100 indications for medical usage of apple cider vinegar. I highly recommend reading Dr. Paul Bragg's *Apple Cider Vinegar, Miracle Health System.* You may understand why I think apple cider vinegar might be the forgotten ancient remedy for the Holy Grail of the fountain of youth! You don't have to travel to the remote Himalaya Mountains or the Pacific Islands for the pursuit of the fountain of youth. Go to the nearest health food store and start with organic apple cider vinegar.

Cholesterol Therapy Based on Compromised Science

This article was published with "My Apology for Telling You the Truth" added to the title.

ॐ ॐ ॐ

During a patient's first visit, I frequently take them off their cholesterol-lowering medications. I often hear them protest that, "My doctor said those medications are for my heart. I may get a heart attack if I stop those medications."

I have to apologize to my patient and the concerned family members. I do not want to contradict their doctor's recommendations nor add to their stress and confusion. However, they need to know the whole story of cholesterol and cholesterol therapy based on "compromised science."

Recommended "normal cholesterol level" guidelines have varied over the years. They suddenly changed 25 years ago, following the now-famous Framingham Heart Study. My 1981 laboratory reference book listed normal cholesterol level range for age 50 at 150-310 mg/dL. Currently, cholesterol over 200 is considered too high for all age groups.

The latest new federal guidelines from the National Cholesterol Education Program focus on lowering LDL, which is considered the main "bad cholesterol." If we follow the new guideline, over 40 million American citizens will fall into the statin drug category, which translates into multibillions of dollars in drug sales and costs to consumers.

The real question is: Who benefits? Do cholesterol-lowering medications really help patients? If not, who benefits from the sudden change in the latest recommendations? So, what really happened? Unknown to the majority of the public, most of the experts on the panel for The National Cholesterol Education Program, which sets the federal guidelines and recommendations for physicians, were on the payroll of the pharmaceutical companies that make statin drugs.

The interpretation of the data and the recommendations for cholesterol treatment are highly compromised by that fact alone. Most physicians are not aware of this "compromised study." However, they are compelled to follow the new guidelines for hypercholesterolemia. They are compelled to recommend a low-fat diet, exercise, and to prescribe statin drugs, which are considered standard medical care.

Lowering the cholesterol for the sake of lowering the cholesterol level does not make any sense at all. Lowering the cholesterol has been associated with violent death, strokes, premature death for elderly patients, and no significant change in overall mortality. Additional side effects of lowering cholesterol include memory loss, amnesia, neuropathy, and depression.

The Framingham Heart Study concluded that a "clear and positive" relationship exists between high cholesterol and heart disease. However, this correlation may not be as strong as indicated in the report because many patients with normal cholesterol also develop heart disease.

C-reactive protein, homocysteine, and lipoprotein-(a) plus the cholesterol may give a better prediction for subsequent cardiovascular problems than the cholesterol level alone. Heavy-metal toxicity and hidden dental infections are also sources of chronic inflammation and cardiovascular problems. The basic science does not support the current broad guidelines for cholesterol treatment nor the recommendations for the general population if the individual does not have other risk factors.

A major downfall of the current recommendations is that a low-fat diet, which usually means a high-carbohydrate diet, leads to insulin resistance, elevated triglycerides, weight gain, and an increase in LDL, while simultaneously lowering HDL, the good cholesterol. Most people do not exercise enough, which alone would improve their metabolism, and lower their cholesterol. Therefore, the only treatment seems to be to resort to using medications to meet the new guidelines.

There are many nutritional supplements that can help lower cholesterol, decrease the viscosity of the blood, improve blood flow, and reduce inflammation. The most well-known natural remedies are fish oil, garlic, niacin, policosanol, red yeast rice extract, Vitamin C, and E, flaxseed, oats, and guggul extract.

A gallbladder/liver flush is an excellent body cleansing program that can support a favorable cholesterol level. It can also support a favorable LDL to HDL cholesterol ratio depending on the individual. You should also remove dental infections and heavy metals from your body. You can also increase your body's metabolism and thyroid activity with kelp, iodine/iodide, and thyroid glandular extracts, all of which can help support a favorable cholesterol level and ratio.

No matter how much I try to explain the above to my patients, I often get phone calls from concerned family members. They repeat their cardiologists' or primary care physicians' highly emotion-charged statements concerning stopping the statin drugs. I sometimes get caught in the crossfire between the patient, who is sincerely seeking alternatives to drug "solutions," and the combined forces of their medical doctor and their concerned family members.

I recommend that you investigate the cholesterol controversy on your own. I hope you can see the cholesterol treatment fallacy without adding more confusion or stress to your life. If you need more detailed information, look for *The Cholesterol Myths* by Uffe Ravnskov, M.D., Ph.D., Dr. Joseph Mercola's cholesterol guidelines at www. mercola.com, and Dr. Duane Graveline's books and articles at www. spacedoc.net.

If you are too concerned about stopping your medication, at least take 200 to 300 mg of coenzyme Q10 per day to counteract the side effects of statin drugs. The co-Q10 will protect you from developing muscle aches, fatigue, cardiomyopathy, or exacerbation of congestive heart failure. Also, implement an individualized nutrition program. Lastly, gradually taper the medication to the lowest dose that is acceptable to your physician.

Fats—Good Fat, Bad Fat, and Killer Fat

I wrote this article to help clear up the confusion about fats that are one of the most complicated topics in nutrition.

ੴ ੴ ੴ

America lives in constant fear of fat as though fats are villains. We are afraid of eating fat, and we end up becoming fatter than ever. Most Americans are grossly misinformed about nutrition, in general, and about the importance of fat and essential fatty acid intake in our diet. We end up eating more of the wrong fats. It is important for us to distinguish good, bad, and killer fats, and to recognize when the good fat becomes a bad fat, and finally becomes a killer fat.

There are two essential fatty acids—Omega-3 and Omega-6—that are vital to good health and must be acquired from food. What are the major symptoms of essential fatty acid deficiency? Omega-3 deficiency symptoms include: growth retardation, weakness, impaired vision, learning disability, tingling sensations in the arms and legs, behavioral changes, hypertension, high triglycerides, inflammation, edema and dry skin, and impaired metabolic and immune function. Omega-6 deficiency symptoms include: eczema, loss of hair, liver and kidney degeneration, excessive thirst, failure of wound healing, sterility in males, miscarriage in females, arthritic pain, growth retardation, and cardiovascular problems.

Fat, protein, and carbohydrates are the major building blocks of nutrients for our body (referred to as "macronutrients"). Omega-3 and -6 fats and eight amino acids from protein are considered "essential." These are not manufactured by the body so they must be acquired from our food. Carbohydrates are needed for energy and acquired from starch and glucose, but carbohydrates are not considered essential nutrients. For example, Eskimos have survived on blubber (fat) and fish protein—almost exclusively without carbohydrates.

Fats can be divided into two major groups: saturated and unsaturated fat. Our body utilizes saturated fats from animals and cholesterol. Saturated fats are involved in all of our known metabolic, immunological, and neurological systems. Saturated fats include butter, coconut, palm, cocoa butter, peanuts, and animal fat.

Unsaturated fats attract oxygen, help generate bioelectrical currents, and help transform bioelectrical energy into cell membranes, muscles, and nerve impulses. Unsaturated fats are metabolically unstable and rapidly oxidize. They need a whole group of antioxidants to regulate their oxidation rate. Unsaturated fats and essential fatty acids, in conjunction with saturated fats, proteins, and glucose, create electrical potentials and build cell membranes as well as hormones.

Two main essential fatty acids (EFAs) can be divided into Omega-3 and Omega-6 unsaturated fats. Major sources of Omega-3 EFAs are: 1) alpha-linolenic acid found in flax seed, canola, soy, walnuts, and green vegetables and 2) eicosapentaenoic acid (EPA) and docosahexaenoic acid (DHA) found in cold water fish like salmon and mackerel.

Major sources of Omega-6 EFAs are: 1) linoleic acid found in safflower, sunflower, soy, walnuts, sesame, pumpkin, and flax seeds, 2) gamma-linolenic acid in borage, evening primrose, and black currant oil, and 3) arachidonic acid found in meats and other animal products.

Monounsaturated Omega-9 fat, which is not considered an EFA but is helpful to the body, comes from olive, almond, avocado, peanut, pecan, cashew, and macadamia oils. There are many different kinds of fats available commercially, but these will not be discussed due to space limitations.

If these essential fatty acids are so essential for our survival and optimum wellness, what are optimal daily doses, how long does it take for these fats to go bad, and how do some turn into "killer fats?"

The daily requirement of EFAs varies by individual depending on body mass, physical activity, stress, and one's emotional state. Most Americans consume adequate amounts of Omega-6 fats. If you are in good health, as a general rule, I recommend one tablespoon daily of Omega-3 from fish and/or flax seed oil. If you are an athlete or are suffering from chronic medical conditions, you may need to double or triple this amount of fish and flax seed oil. I like to use fish oil, especially cod liver oil, and flax seed oils, since they are widely available and easy to use. However, you may use the other oils mentioned above. Walnuts are an excellent source of Omega-3 and Omega-6 fats.

Any oils and fats that have been processed or hydrogenated, or partially hydrogenated, like soy oil, corn oil, shortening, or margarine, are high in "trans-fatty acids." These are considered bad fats, very unhealthy, and should be avoided. There are many hidden hydrogenated or partially hydrogenated oils in all processed foods, such as cookies, donuts, salad dressings, chips, etc. Avoid fried or deep fried food. In addition, high levels of carbohydrates and sugar in the diet can raise triglycerides.

The worst combination is a diet that is high in carbohydrates, sugar, and hydrogenated trans fats. This combination will eventually even transform good fats into bad fats and eventually, in the absence of proper vitamins, antioxidants, and minerals, turn bad fats into a gang of killer fats.

Folk Remedy From Russia: Oil Therapy by Dr. Karach

When I wrote this article, I referred to sunflower seed oil and peanut oil. Since then, sesame seed oil has become my favorite oil to use in a practice known as "oil pulling." All three oils work in this very effective folk remedy from Russia.

꿀 꿀 꿀

Folk remedies have an endearing quality for mankind because they are simple, easy to use, and often effective. The most well-known folk remedies are garlic and apple cider vinegar, which I have mentioned in this chapter. In Russia, garlic is considered to be an antibiotic comparable to penicillin in America.

Chicken soup for colds and duct tape for warts are other well-known folk remedies. What about oil therapy? This is not some exotic aromatic oil, but an oil that you can buy at your local grocery store.

This lesser-known folk remedy called oil therapy was introduced by Dr. Karach, a medical doctor from Russia. Karach presented a paper to the All-Ukranian Association of the Academy of Science of the USSR and explained an unusual, simple healing process that uses cold-pressed seed oils.

The exciting factor of this oil therapy is its simplicity. It consists of swishing cold-pressed seed oil in the mouth. The healing process is accomplished by extracting toxic waste without disturbing the healthy microflora. Dr. Karash says humans are living only half of their potential life span. They could potentially live to be 140 to 150 years old by simply following his oil therapy.

Dr. Karach claims oil therapy is effective for the following conditions: headache, bronchitis, lung and liver conditions, toothache, thrombosis, blood disorders, arthritis, paralysis, eczema, gastric ulcers, intestinal disorders, heart and kidney conditions, encephalitis, nervous conditions, and female disorders.

The best oil to use is cold-pressed sunflower oil or peanut oil. In the morning before breakfast, on an empty stomach, place one tablespoon in the mouth but do not swallow it. Slowly swish the oil in the mouth and through the teeth for 20 minutes.

As the oil is swished in the mouth, it becomes mixed with saliva. Chewing activates enzymes, and enzymes draw toxins out of the blood. The oil must not be swallowed because it becomes toxic. There is a noticeable change in the appearance of the oil. It gets thinner and turns white. It is then spit from the mouth into the sink or toilet.

If the oil is still yellow, it has not been swished thoroughly or long enough. After the oil has been removed from the mouth, rinse with warm water, mixed with a half teaspoon of sea salt and baking soda—several times. Then, brush the gums and tongue with salt and baking soda. If you have chronic sinusitis, you may also sniff up the mixture of salt and baking soda to clean the nasal and sinus passages.

If Dr. Karach is correct, this simple oil therapy is preventive as well as curative. He states, "With the use of this therapy, I healed my chronic blood disease of 15 years. I was healed within 3 days of an acute arthritis that forced me to lie in bed."

I found an article written by Dr. Karach while I was reviewing my old conference materials. The date he presented his work in Russia is unknown. I have been emphasizing the complexity of dental/medical problems that have been related to so many unexplained medical conditions.

I believe Dr. Karach's oil therapy is a simple and elegant way to solve common dental-related medical problems. This oil therapy is also an excellent dental hygiene self-care therapy. Your visits to your dentist and medical doctor will be less frequent. After all, I never enjoyed going to the dentist. For that matter, it's even worse to be evaluated by a medical doctor. I recommend that all my patients follow Dr. Karach's regimen. Thank you, Dr. Karach! This is a gift of love from Russia!

Notes

12

Holistic Medical Articles

*Chronic disease is associated
with a loss of voltage and a
reversal of polarity in cells.*

- Fritz Albert Popp

Holistic medicine recognizes that health and healing depend on the treatment of the entire person. In conventional medicine, this is difficult because doctors specialize in and become experts at treating compartmentalized portions of the body.

Quantum medicine is on the fringes of holistic medicine—and about as far from conventional medicine as you can possibly get. Energy medicine, that is a major theme in this book, fits within quantum medicine more than any other branch of holistic medicine.

It is important for patients to realize the differences between holistic and conventional medicine—and understand that "quantum" introduces electrical concepts that are far outside either of these methodologies. Most medical doctors have no understanding of quantum physics, let alone its application in medicine. In his book, *Biology of Belief*, former medical school professor, Dr. Bruce Lipton, relays how he accidentally discovered the connection between quantum physics and biology when he bought Heinz Pagels' *The Cosmic Code: Quantum Physics As the Language of Nature* at an airport.

Energy medicine cannot be entirely explained, but neither can quantum physics. From ancient Greece onward, science has searched for a description of physical reality. At the beginning of the 20th century (around 1900), physics saw matter as discrete particles with both gravitational mass and electrical charge properties. However, as quantum physics evolved and subatomic particles were discovered, physicists had to confront unexplained phenomena. Subatomic particles that they observed disappeared suddenly from a starting point and, as if by magic, appeared somewhere else. Disappearing particles are not the only mystery in quantum physics. Particles sometimes act like waves, and waves sometimes act like particles. From approximately 1930 onward, physicists simply had to deal with unanswered questions concerning particles and waves.

Unfortunately, not all branches of science are as tolerant of unexplained phenomena as quantum physics. Medicine, or at least conventional medicine, resists anything that cannot be explained. If physicists can cope with paradoxes, why can't doctors?

In this chapter, I have collected a number of my favorite articles that cover various topics in holistic medicine.

Combat Medical Care and Holistic Medicine

At the time that I wrote this article, I was a medical officer in the U.S. Army Reserves. I have recently retired, and I plan to devote the extra time to work on my book, as well as medical conferences, to share what I have learned with other physicians. Readers may check my Web site for updates on both of these projects (preventionandhealing.com).

એ એ એ

Our nation is at war with terrorism. If you are an American soldier in the middle of a combat zone, the last thing you need is a holistic medical doctor taking care of you. You need a highly trained combat medic and trauma surgeon to control hemorrhage and secure your airway from blasts or ballistic injuries.

I have been a medical officer in the U.S. Army Reserve for over 20 years and currently serve as a chief medical officer with the 301st Combat Support Hospital (CSH) in St. Louis. As part of my Reserve duty, I served with the 67th CSH over 2 years ago in Germany. Combat medical care and holistic medicine seem mutually exclusive, on opposite ends of the spectrum of medicine, but I believe they can be closely intertwined.

Combat medical care is for acute, heroic, emergency medical care to save lives from trauma. Holistic medicine is for preventive and post-surgical care following crisis management as well as treatment of chronic illness. Successful care for soldiers can be achieved by integrating the expedient surgical intervention and holistic postsurgical care, which I call the Army's way of holistic medicine.

I recently came back from Ft. Sam Houston after completing training on Advanced Trauma Life Support and Combat Casualty Care. Military medical training was mentally and physically demanding under the harsh realistic combat-like conditions where the medical officers were challenged by caring for wounded soldiers under fire. I have great respect for those highly motivated young health care officers, medical doctors, dentists, nurses, physicians' assistants and nurse practitioners from all three branches of the Armed Services.

Why do I mention holistic medicine in combat medical care? Because some of the most common reasons why soldiers are not "combat ready" are due to medical illness and combat stress. The Army recognizes that vector-born diseases from sand fly fever, leishmaniasis, or combat stress are just as destructive and disabling of the soldier's strength as trauma from a blast or gunshot wound. Our training not only included advanced trauma life support but also training in operational entomology, preventive medicine, combat epidemiology, high-risk infectious disease for military operations, combat stress control, and chaplain's services. When you add all these multidisciplinary fields, it becomes more like the Army's version of holistic medicine.

If we can imagine the war as a symbol of disease like cancer or a heart attack disabling our body, then we can make a dramatic declaration of war on cancer or heart disease. But chaos and misunderstanding soon begin, and the first casualty of war is the truth. The truth is that in real life we should not treat symptoms with pharmaceutical drugs or surgery when other options exist.

There are times in real life when combat medical care, such as surgery, intubations, radiation, and chemotherapy may be required for acute crisis management. But a far superior approach is to focus on prevention and holistic approach—building our body's immune system through proper diet, nutrition, and detoxification.

The best preventive medicine on the battlefield is fire power superiority. Real life is not a combat field. And, unlike the combat field where a quick fix is urgently needed, in real life we need to explore the underlying causes of illnesses. We need to assess why someone got sick at all. For example, five of the most neglected areas of assessment by medical professionals are environmental toxicity, allergies, parasites, hidden dental problems, and nutritional deficiencies. When we integrate the many disciplines of the medical fields, we can truly restore our immune systems to handle the enemy, whether it is a virus, parasite, heavy metal, or hidden infection, and prevent the next "war," i.e., disease.

Hypoglycemia: The Great Masquerader

Hypoglycemia has historically been much more recognized by alternative medicine practitioners than traditional physicians. It is also one of the most feared complications of either Type I or Type II diabetes. According to a study by International Diabetes Federation, the number of people around the world with diabetes has skyrocketed in the last two decades (from 30 million to 230 million). There has been an increase in both Type I and Type II diabetes.

Here is my article about hypoglycemia that was published in the St. Louis *Healthy Planet* magazine:

ᶳ᷿ ᶳ᷿ ᶳ᷿

If you are suffering from frequent headaches, irritability, mood swings, poor concentration, sugar cravings, weakness, or anxiety, you might be suffering from unsuspected hypoglycemia. Other symptoms include sweating, visual disturbance, extreme hunger, palpitation and rapid heart rate, syncope (brief loss of consciousness), seizures, and irrational behavior.

Chemically, hypoglycemia is defined as a blood sugar level of less than 50 milligrams/deciliter (mg/dL) and is not always symptomatic. True chemical hypoglycemia, based on a blood test, is not common, except in diabetic patients on diabetic medications or insulin. However, mild hypoglycemia and sugar cravings are an epidemic health threat in industrialized countries.

Eating refined, super-sized, and nutrient-depleted food often triggers more sugar cravings, insulin regulation problems, and obesity. After eating a high caloric, "empty" meal, lethargy and hypoglycemia follow. For susceptible individuals, the multitude of hypoglycemic symptoms masquerade with a wrong diagnosis, such as migraine headaches, candidiasis, anxiety, or panic disorder, and are followed by an inappropriate treatment.

A glucose tolerance test, performed in a physician's office, is a medical test designed to rule out glucose intolerance and hypoglycemia, as well as screen for pre-diabetic conditions. However, the test uses a high dose of glucose and often overlooks many sugar-sensitive patients who react to only minor changes in blood glucose levels. Seizures, syncope, and extreme irrational behavior can be triggered in highly sensitive individuals with only moderate blood sugar fluctuations.

Diet and a nutritional supplement program is the basic foundation for controlling hypoglycemia and its related symptoms. All refined sugar and carbohydrates, including fruit juices and honey, should be eliminated from the diet. Eat high-protein snacks between meals. Follow a low-carbohydrate diet, such as the Zone Diet by Barry Sears, Ph.D., or the South Beach Diet by Arthur Agatston, M.D.

The Zone Diet or the South Beach Diet are good starting points for the majority of the population who are susceptible to hypoglycemia with insulin sensitivity. Nutritional supplements should include digestive enzymes, B-complex vitamins, and a full spectrum of antioxidants and trace minerals, especially chromium and vanadium. *Gymnema* leaf extract has been used effectively for hypoglycemia and pre-diabetic conditions.

Liver and adrenal dysfunctions, rather than pancreas and insulin disregulations, are some of the most common hidden culprits causing sugar cravings and hypoglycemia. Mineral imbalances—especially calcium, magnesium, sodium, and potassium, as well as a chromium deficiency—set the conditions for sugar sensitivity. Caffeinated beverages, alcohol, food allergies, and hidden infections can also exacerbate sugar problems. Hypoglycemia and sugar cravings are some of the most common symptoms I see in my practice. They disguise several other physical complaints and are often ignored or mistreated. Hypoglycemia is truly a great masquerader.

Asthma: Are We Missing Something?

The Centers for Disease Control (CDC) says that "asthma is a prevalent chronic illness in the United States that has been increasing in prevalence since 1980." Asthma, like diabetes, may also be related to worldwide environmental pollution and mercury exposure. Taurine, one of the body's sulfur-containing amino acids that is vulnerable to mercury poisoning, protects the kidneys, retina, liver, heart, and lungs from free radical damage by toxic metals.

The alarming news about the increased incidence of asthma prompted me to ask, "Are we missing something?"

&a &a &a

Asthma is a disease of the airway. It is characterized by inflammatory hyper-responsiveness that manifests clinically in shortness of breath and wheezing. It is also sometimes associated with cough and chest tightness. Asthma has become one of the fastest-growing causes of medical disability and morbidity for all ages, but especially for the young in industrialized countries.

Asthma may manifest as an acute attack or chronic exacerbations. The attacks are often triggered by: 1) exposure to irritants, such as smoke, pollen, and cold air, 2) allergens, such as dust, mold, animal dander, air pollution, and petrochemical products, or 3) bronchial or sinus infection. Acid reflux, viral infection, congestive heart failure, foreign body, or drug reaction are also common conditions associated with recurrent asthma. However, there is a large portion of people suffering from no obvious triggering agents or infections. These individuals are not responding to conventional therapy. Are we missing something?

Standard treatment for asthma typically consists of bronchodilators, such as albuterol and corticosteroids in the form of oral, nasal, or intravenous preparations. There are many other forms of medications for asthma, including cromolyn sodium, leukotriene antagonists like Singulair, theophylline, and the new generation of long-acting bronchodilators.

Despite aggressive usage of multiple medications for the management of asthma, more than 15 million Americans are suffering. Over 5,000 die from severe asthma attacks every year. The total medical costs related to asthma are estimated at over 14 billion dollars. The overall rate of asthma and the resulting financial burden have been rising for the last 30 years. Are we missing something?

According to James Braly, M.D., expert on food allergies, wheat, milk, and eggs are among the most likely foods that will trigger an asthma attack. Corn, soy, and peanuts are also common foods that can exacerbate asthma. Food coloring and preservatives are also unsuspected triggering agents. Food allergy tests and a rotational diet of foods are essential parts of managing asthma.

Some of the natural remedies for asthma include nettle (*Urtica dioica*), mullein, ephedra, licorice root (*Glycyrrhiza*), cayenne pepper, and intestinal cleansers to remove the mucous buildup in the small and large intestines. Hydration with plenty of water is also essential. Avoiding mucous-forming foods, especially grains and dairy products, is also critical to the proper management of asthma.

Two of the most unsuspected cases of asthma in my clinical experience have been resolved by treating a hidden dental infection and a parasite infection. These two overlooked areas are a lot more common than you may think as causative factors of a variety of illnesses. In asthma, they can provoke an inflammatory response.

As an example, a 45-year-old female developed life-threatening asthma 6 months after she had a root canal procedure. She had been in and out of the hospital with one crisis after another for asthma attacks. She was not responding to medications or natural remedies until her asymptomatic infected root canal tooth was extracted. Another case involved a 60-year-old farmer's wife with over 30 years of frequent asthma attacks. Two rounds of parasite medications allowed her to become totally free from recurrent asthma attacks.

Other alternative therapies to consider include acupuncture, acupressure massage therapy, spinal adjustments by an experienced chiropractor, and the Buteyko Method for controlling asthma. The Buteyko Method was developed by Konstantin Pavlovich Buteyko from Russia. It includes training in a technique for deliberate shallow breathing and carbon dioxide regulation. It is worth investigating. Therapists who specialize in the Buteyko Method for asthma may be located with an Internet search.

One of my favorite therapies is an injection technique called infraspinatous respiratory response (IRR) therapy, developed by Harry H. Philibert, M.D., from Louisiana. Asthma patients often have an asymptomatic painful area by the shoulder blades called the infraspinatous muscle. Injecting local anesthetics like lidocaine or procaine at the trigger points for IRR can sometimes invoke a dramatic response for asthma relief.

In summary, asthma has become a very common debilitating medical epidemic in the United States for all ages with increased morbidity and mortality. A significant portion of asthma sufferers do not respond to conventional medical treatments. The more we use bronchodilator medications or corticosteroids, the more side effects and mortality occur.

It is time for us to reevaluate asthma medical management. It is time for us to ask the question, "Are we missing something?" We must look far beyond common infections and allergens. Consider hidden parasite infections or dental infections. Consider other forms of alternative medical therapies as mentioned above. Sometimes, the response can be dramatic and almost miraculous.

Hypothyroidism: Unsuspected Cause for Fatigue and Obesity

Hypothyroidism is another example of a condition that has historically been much more recognized by alternative medicine practitioners than traditional physicians. Alternative medical practitioners understand that blood tests for thyroid depend on a feedback mechanism in the pituitary gland that is often poisoned by heavy metals. They also understand that the health of the thyroid may involve more than just hormone production that is tracked with blood tests. For example, the minerals that the body needs for thyroid health may be analyzed with a hair analysis test that is not used in conventional medicine. My article on hypothyroidism, written for the *Healthy Planet* magazine, describes a holistic approach to caring for the thyroid gland.

≈ ≈ ≈

Mild, subclinical hypothyroidism (lower than normal thyroid activity) is one of the most common medical conditions associated with fatigue, obesity, and many other illnesses. Yet, hypothyroidism is often not recognized and, therefore, not treated by most medical professionals.

Dr. Broda Barnes, M.D., devoted his life's work to the study of the thyroid gland. He boldly states, "At least 40 percent of the American people have hypothyroidism and suffer from fatigue and obesity." This is needless suffering since inexpensive natural thyroid glandulars are widely available; many people are suffering from the consequence of lack of medical knowledge and undertreatment by their medical doctors.

There are many faces of thyroid deficiency beyond fatigue and obesity. As with most illnesses or combinations of symptoms, there are usually multiple causes. If all causes are not resolved, then one may improve, but optimum health may never be achieved. Thyroid deficiency may be a contributing factor in all of the following: morning sluggishness, cold hands and feet, cold intolerance, proneness to all kinds of infections, arthritis and rheumatisms, migraine headaches, eczema, psoriasis, acne, depression, menstrual problems, infertility, diabetes, hypoglycemia, hypertension, fluid retentions, hypercholesterolemia, heart attack, narcolepsy, insomnia, and accelerated aging.

If hypothyroidism is so common, why isn't your doctor able to detect it from the blood thyroid function test (T3, T4, and TSH). Unfortunately, the blood thyroid tests often show a normal range. Medical doctors usually rely solely on these blood tests for thyroid function, while ignoring a patient's clinical symptoms.

Short of obvious severe hypothyroidism, Dr. Broda Barnes states the most reliable indication of thyroid function is the basal temperature test, not the blood thyroid function test. Diagnosis for mild, subclinical hypothyroidism is determined when: 1) the blood test for thyroid function is normal or low normal range, 2) the patient is complaining of fatigue with many other symptoms as described above, and 3) he/she has low basal body temperature. In addition, to aid in determination of your thyroid activity at the cellular level, an analysis can be made of the body composition of hair tissue mineral content of calcium, magnesium, sodium and potassium levels, and their ratios to each other.

A description of how to take your basal temperature can be found on my Web site at www.preventionandhealing.com.

Thyroid gland enzymes need many minerals, such as iodine, selenium, zinc, and iron, to function at optimal level for the production of thyroid hormones (T4) and to convert to biologically active thyroid hormone (T3). These enzymes are highly sensitive to toxic metals, especially mercury. The causes for epidemic proportions of mild, subclinical hypothyroidism are complex and alarming. Dental disorders, especially silver-mercury amalgams, are one of the commonly overlooked, yet controversial, issues associated with hypothyroidism.

Once hypothyroidism is determined by low basal temperature, blood tests, and a clinical-symptom survey, the treatment plan must reflect an individualized, holistic approach, rather than the usual knee-jerk reaction—prescribing synthetic thyroid medications. A majority of my patients respond better to a therapeutic trial of natural thyroid glandulars, such as Armour Thyroid, rather than levothyroxine. The natural thyroid glandular supplementation is widely available and inexpensive. Often, hypothyroid patients need concurrent adrenal glandular support.

In addition to thyroid support, a holistic approach to resolving hypothyroidism would include several other elements. The individual should start with a basic body detoxification program. A dietary program, including an analysis of food allergies along with a nutritional program of vitamins and minerals, is the cornerstone to the rejuvenation of one's health. The dietary and nutritional programs should be specific to the individual as determined by appropriate tests.

These steps may be followed with more targeted detoxification programs, such as the use of chelation therapy for heavy-metal toxicity, again as determined by individual testing. Additional considerations may include replacement of silver-mercury amalgams with safer, nonallergenic, nontoxic dental materials as determined and accomplished by an experienced biological dentist.

Identifying and resolving hypothyroidism as a contributing factor to fatigue and obesity, as well a myriad of other illnesses, may help you accomplish the "last step" to achieving optimum health.

Notes

13

Integrating Internal Medicine With Alternative/Complementary Medicine

Cure sometimes, treat often, comfort always.

- Hippocrates

The *Merriam-Webster Dictionary* defines the verb "integrate" as "forming, coordinating, or blending into a functioning or unified whole." In medicine, nearly everyone is in favor of blending conventional therapies with alternatives—except for those whose income is tied to so-called "scientific medicine." The critics who call integrative medicine a "fad" often ignore the fact that there is a public demand for alternative treatments. A landmark study done in 1993 showed that 1 in 3 Americans have used an alternative therapy, often under the "medical radar."

While my practice may not reflect the classic model of integrative care due to the fact that I use energy medicine for evaluations, the health care that I provide also uses the word "complementary" to help patients understand that the treatments are used *with conventional medicine* and not as replacements or alternatives.

In this chapter, I have presented articles that provide readers with examples of how I treat the whole person—and not a disease.

Chest Pain Rituals: What is Chest Pain, Anyway?

Heart disease used to be the #1 killer in the United States. In 2005, the American Cancer Society reported that cancer kills more Americans under 85 than heart disease. The International Agency for Research on Cancer has also projected that cancer will be the leading cause of death worldwide in 2010.

This article, written for St. Louis' *Healthy Planet* magazine, describes the rituals of conventional medicine that convince patients with chest pain that they have had a heart attack.

ða ða ða

What would you do if you're over 50 years old and experience chest pain and shortness of breath in the middle of the night? This can be an extremely frightening experience. "Heart attack" is the first thing that may come to your mind. People over the age of 50 have been programmed to react to chest pain with suspicions of a heart problem and heart attack ("acute coronary syndrome" is the new terminology for chest pain). This is the beginning of the ritual of allopathic medicine.

Your first step is to go to the nearest hospital emergency room to rule out heart attack. Due to tremendous pressure over a potential malpractice suit, the emergency room physicians will subject you to a ritual of test after test to diagnose the probable cause of your chest pain. If you have any minor changes in EKG or blood lab test results, most people over 50 years old will automatically be admitted to the hospital to rule out heart attack.

In the hospital, you will be hooked to electronic monitoring. You will go through a cascade of more tests and procedures. I won't bore you with the details. After the cardiac catherization, it is not uncommon to hear that you have 80-90% occlusion in the artery of your heart.

The doctors will typically recommend cardiac angioplasty, placement of one or more stents, or a bypass operation. You may be told, "If you don't have an angioplasty or a bypass, you may have a full-blown heart attack and drop dead any moment." Next thing you know, you are on the operating table.

One of my patients, over time, had seven cardiac angioplasty procedures, plus a valve replacement, and a bypass operation. Another patient recently had four stents placed for critically occluded heart vessels, but still has chest pain. Another patient had two bypass operations. The doctors told him they can't do any more operations. The patient is still suffering from chest pain while on a maximum dose of heart medication. Is there a missing link between chest pain and procedures like angioplasty, stent placements, and bypass operations?

Western medicine analyzes the human body from a mechanical point of view. If you have chest pain and an angiogram shows 95% occlusion of the coronary artery, the doctors assume that you have chest pain as a result of the occlusion of the artery. They also assume the occlusion is cutting off the blood supply to the heart. The most logical thing to do by cardiologists and cardiothoracic surgeons is to open up the blocked blood vessel by angioplasty, stent placement, and/or bypass operation.

But what happens to that logic when the patient continues to experience chest pain, even after angioplasty, stent placement, or a bypass operation? One recent possibility for an explanation of non-cardiac chest pain is "acid reflux." The patient will be put on antacid medication for the rest of his or her life after an extensive gastrointestinal (GI) evaluation by a GI specialist.

What does the doctor do if the patient continues to have chest pain after stent placements or a bypass operation and is on a maximum dose of heart medication and antacid medication? A "difficult" patient will be put on antianxiety medication for suspected anxiety and stress-related chest pain. If the chest pain continues, the next move is referring the patient to a psychiatrist for mind-altering medication to dissociate the patient's body and detach the patient's mind from the chest pain.

This tragic scenario will repeat for millions of people. For every step we take, there are cumulative side effects stemming from the invasive procedures and medications.

While I was on active duty for the U.S. Army a few years ago, a 38-year-old Master Sergeant came to see me with complaints of chest pain. He had extensive cardiac and GI evaluations. Every test came back negative. I gave this particular soldier, whose career was on the line, a trigger-point injection on his right shoulder blade and a specific tender area on his spine (the para-vertebral area at T-4) for a pinched nerve. His chest pain resolved in one minute. His military career was saved from a medical discharge for unexplained chest pain.

Another patient's chest pain was resolved by extraction of an infected tooth. Still another patient responded to nutritional therapy and chelation therapy. In addition, some people appear to have a perfect heart condition and still suffer from a massive heart attack due to an emotional shock or grief.

So, it is time to reevaluate "chest pain rituals." What is chest pain, anyway? I believe chest pain is like any other pain in the body and can be evaluated from a holistic view of mind/body/spirit. We should think of the human body not only from a biomechanical and biochemical view, but also as a bioenergetic phenomenon.

When there is blocked energy flow, the disturbance of the flow of energy will create pain. This pain can often be corrected with nutrition (biochemistry), acupuncture, or emotional release (both bioenergetic). Invasive procedures like angioplasty, stent placement, and bypass operations can be used as a last resort, not as a first attempt.

In summary, when you experience chest pain in the middle of the night, don't panic. You should go to the hospital immediately and follow through with the rituals of allopathic medicine. However, don't submit to invasive procedures like stent placement or a bypass operation immediately. Explore other preventive and alternative therapies before thinking about a stent placement or a bypass operation.

Forbidden Miracle Cures: Paradox of Alternative Medicine

If you are searching for a cure for some chronic disease, you will not find it in conventional or alternative medicine—and for different reasons. Conventional medicine seeks to *manage an illness* rather than cure it. Alternative/complementary medicine is burdened with so many claims of miracle remedies that it becomes almost impossible for a patient to sort out what works and what does not. In this article, I explain some of the dangers of alternative/complementary medicine.

ॐ ॐ ॐ

Claiming "cure" for any chronic illness, especially cancer, has been a thorny issue for medical doctors for many years. However, you will hear many so-called "alternative/complementary" medical practitioners (many of them without a license to practice or with a mail order diploma) who are eager to claim a cure for cancer, heart disease, diabetes, osteoporosis, arthritis, Alzheimer's, pain, and more.

When you combine the seductive words "forbidden," "secret," or "miracle" with cures, it becomes a powerful selling tool. It has a compelling allure of magical healing remedies. These words have often been combined with those "ancient lost" herbs or fruit drinks from the Tibetan mountains or remote islands. It's good for marketing and business promotion, but do these "cures" really work?

Every day, some of my patients bring the latest seductive advertisements claiming new cures for their conditions. Either they've started on new cures or wanted my blessing to try them. As a rule, I do not oppose my patients' desires to try new alternative therapies, unless I feel individuals are too frail and the therapies may endanger his/her condition.

My medical practice integrates internal medicine with alternative/complementary medicine. I'm overwhelmed by vast amounts of new information, especially from all the hyped "forbidden, miracle cures."

Sometimes, I think the hyped "new alternative cure" claims in newsletters and magazines are far worse and misleading than the slick TV commercials by the big pharmaceutical companies.

Anyway, I always remind my patients that, while they may try the newest, latest alternative therapy, not to forget my core recommendations—basic body cleansing and heavy-metal detoxification, an individualized diet including the elimination of food allergies, and fixing dental problems with a biological dentist. Chiropractic adjustment, massage therapy, or psychological counseling are also very important parts of the healing process for body/mind connections.

Too often, I observe temporary improvement of symptoms for my patients without long-lasting benefits. Some people will spend thousands of dollars on hyped network marketing nutritional supplements when it is not indicated. It may not be bad for them, but they might be wasting their time and money on actions that divert them from addressing their more serious medical problems.

Once in a while, a patient will deteriorate rapidly. Eventually, I usually find out that they have stopped my regimen and only followed the "forbidden" or "miracle" cure therapy. One of these is the Rife frequency generator. This device has been known to "cure all diseases." Many people are silently suffering from side effects.

There is nothing wrong with the original Rife frequency generator. The problems occur because many models in the market are imitations of the original Rife frequency generator. The manufacturers of the immitations claim their products are the same as the original when they aren't.

Most people, even if they had the proper equipment, don't have medical training or proper intructions to use the equipment. For very sick and frail patients, it's like playing "Russian roulette."

I'm not trying to scare you from trying the newest, latest alternative medical therapies. I want you to be informed, or at least be warned, before the next time you read or hear the latest "forbidden" or "miracle cure" on TV, radio, or in a newsletter.

I've been practicing long enough that I don't get too excited about either hype from the conventional medicine world that touts the latest pharmaceutical products or newly discovered tree barks from a faraway Amazon jungle. If you hear the latest new miracle cure, let me know. I will be the first one to test the product, but I will not abandon my core recommendations.

As far as I'm concerned, there's no such thing as a "forbidden" or "miracle" cure. We can certainly discuss a medical therapy that's been suppressed in the medical literature, but this doesn't necessarily mean it's a "forbidden cure." Blindly following these much-hyped claims may be paradoxically dangerous to your health. Be informed. Healing comes from within.

Cancer and Cancerous Mind: Cancer as a Turning Point

If articles could have a musical theme song, this article's song would be Billy Joel's "Only the Good Die Young" from one of his popular albums in the 1970s. At the time that I wrote this piece, I was overwhelmed by the number of nice people who develop cancer. Strangely, this is still true.

᷂ ᷂ ᷂

Is there such a thing as a cancerous mind or cancer personality? Cancer patients, as a rule, are some of the nicest, decent people you will encounter in your life. I remember Mary, a 75-year-old lady who came to see me with a bronchial cough 20 years ago when I was starting out as a young physician on the staff of a managed care clinic.

I suspected she had bronchitis and started her on antibiotics. She came back several weeks later with a persistent cough. This time, I thought she may have pneumonia. I recommended a chest x-ray (CXR) and put her on a stronger antibiotic. However, she refused the CXR. She was more concerned about me and how managed care comes down on doctors to cut costs. She insisted that she would get better in no time with the stronger antibiotic.

Several weeks later, Mary came back with a cough and hoarseness in her voice. Again, she refused the CXR and seemed more concerned about my working under the pressure of the managed care system. This time I persisted, and the CXR was ordered. The report came back highly suspicious for lung cancer and recommended further evaluation. Mary was sent to a cancer specialist. A few months later, I found out she died while going through chemotherapy.

For the last 20 years, my practice has been gradually transformed from an internal medicine practice to an integrated alternative/complementary medicine practice. During this time, I have seen more cancer patients looking for alternative/complementary medicine. I still find that most cancer patients are some of the nicest, decent people I have encountered in my practice.

Currently, 1 out of 2 men and 1 out of 3 women will develop cancer in their lifetime. One out of 8 women will develop breast cancer during their lifetime. Why are so many nice people developing cancer? Are mean, hot-tempered, aggressive people immune to cancer? Not really. They are more prone to have a heart attack before developing cancer.

In the last 50 years, medical scientists have hypothesized the development of cancer cells based on the influence of Watson Crick's DNA model. Genetic mutation at the DNA level was the suspected cause. Ever since, scientists have been targeting cancer cells with "magic bullets" to make corrections at molecular and genetic levels.

I am not too optimistic that we will ever find a cure by discovering cancer genes (oncogenes) at the genetic level. Scientists have tried for the last 50 years without significant improvement in advanced metastatic cancer.

Instead of the gene, it is time to explore factors that influence genetic expression, called epigenetics. Epigenetics can be environmental toxins, synthetic chemicals and pesticides, infections from viruses, fungus or parasites, specific nutritional deficiencies and, finally, a patient's unresolved emotions and cancerous mind.

Each cancer patient has a unique story to tell. A patient's emotional life history may give us a clue to the development of cancer. A generation of unresolved emotional conflicts will pass on to the next generation in the crystal matrix of DNA.

DNA is not a two-dimensional nucleic acid sequence. The Human Genome Project has sequenced human genome in vain for a two-dimensional sequence of DNA. DNA is a multidimensional crystal matrix. It stores human experiences in a vibrational resonance of the time-warping crystal matrix.

A diagnosis of cancer gives an individual an opportunity, as a turning point, to reexamine and rediscover life. Almost all cancer patients have unresolved emotional conflicts. Most cancer patients always think of other people first before they think about themselves, just like Mary.

There are many books on nutritional therapies and detox programs for cancer. The first step is detoxifying and nourishing your mind. Reclaim your childhood dreams. Let go of your fear, anger, and resentment. Take care of yourself first by forgiving yourself and then others. Start praying. Meditate and laugh. Feed your mind/body with positive, loving thoughts and with healing foods.

I recommend reading *Cancer As a Turning Point: A Handbook for People with Cancer, Their Families, and Health Professionals* by Lawrence LeShan, Ph.D. I also recommend looking for the articles on my Web site at preventionandhealing.com titled "Nutritional Therapies for Cancer" and "Accidental Cure."

Part 4

Patient Success Stories and Testimonials

Notes

14

Conquering Cancer

There are no guarantees in life, but I feel I am now taking positive, proactive steps to maximize my chances that cancer will not return.
E.M. (Patient)

Without real-life clinical experience, medical treatments are just theories. Revelations in medicine arise out of joint discoveries between a physician and his/her patients. While I have been able to shape the general direction of my career with research, clinical outcomes have always offered me the milestones I needed to continue.

Disease is the manifestation of the human body's response to unnatural elements in the environment. The solution is not to modulate human genetics with medication, but to move the toxins out of the way so the body can recover. The modern challenge in medicine involves a relatively quick determination as to which toxins, hidden infections, or related structural problems are creating obstacles to health. My search for an efficient evaluation tool led me to biocybernetic medicine and Dr. Rhinehold Voll's EAV device, which I prefer to call Acupuncture Meridian Assessment (AMA).

This chapter presents patient success stories, and some are in their own words. These case histories have been added for readers and for other doctors who are conducting their own search for an advanced diagnostic tool.

Success Story: Cheryl's Adenocarcinoma of the Lung (Lung Cancer)

Twelve years after Cheryl was diagnosed with adenocarcinoma, she has many interesting stories to tell about her battle with a form of lung cancer that her radiologist told her would be fatal. Statistics tell us that lung cancer is the leading cause of cancer death and that survival past 5 years is extremely rare.

Even though 85 percent of people who have lung cancer are smokers, Cheryl was a healthy, nonsmoker who took care of herself and avoided secondhand smoke. In such cases, conventional medicine refers to air pollution as a risk factor. My clinical experience has helped me identify several other important factors including:

- Biological terrain issues
- Parasites and heavy metals
- Food allergies

Cheryl and most of my patients have all of these factors when they are first evaluated at my clinic.

A Weakened Immune System Cannot Detect Cancer Cells

When the body's immune system is functioning properly, it is programmed to search and destroy unhealthy cells, including cancer cells. When the immune system is weak, this capability breaks down because of stressors that interfere with healthy biochemistry. This can go on for a very long time before any physical symptoms present themselves.

Cheryl Coughed Up Blood But Otherwise Felt Healthy

In May of 1996, Cheryl and her husband were just back from a 12-day trip to Europe when her body gave her a clue that there was something wrong with her lungs. Even though she felt healthy, she coughed up blood in the middle of the night; her husband took her to a hospital emergency room (ER) where she was given a chest x-ray. Her diagnosis:

> *…most likely a broken blood*
> *vessel from a small infection.*

Although a chest X-ray is the most common test performed to detect lung cancer, Cheryl's tumor was not visible and the ER staff missed it completely.

Cheryl's Lowest Point

In the midst of her chemotherapy, Cheryl's mother passed away. Her father had died 15 years before, and the loss of her mother took Cheryl to a very low point emotionally. She felt as though *she* was dying and thought she would soon join her mother. Throughout her ordeal, Cheryl was plagued by questions about her mysterious illness. She felt she had been young and healthy, and she kept asking herself, "How did I get lung cancer?" Somehow Cheryl found the strength to keep going and to keep searching for a way to "fix" her body.

Cheryl's First Visit to My Office

Cheryl remembers that, although she brought some of her medical records with her to my office, she's certain that her paperwork did not contain information about the exact location of her cancer. She was so new to the diagnostic methods that I use, she did not understand the details that an Acupuncture Meridian Assessment and a biological terrain assessment would provide. In her words:

> *When Dr. Yu measured 54 acupuncture points on my hands*
> *and feet, he said, "It's your left lung." My husband and*
> *I looked at each other at that point—and again, when he*
> *asked us if we had fertility issues. He was correct about*

both. He said my body was so acidic that I had the profile of an 82-year-old woman and I was 39 at that time. I learned that I was not digesting protein, and I was highly allergic to dairy—even though I loved dairy. I also had a very high level of mercury, even though I did not have many silver fillings. Everything Dr. Yu said that day made sense. We would work on my cancer by treating the underlying causes. And that's what I have done for the past 11 years.

My Clinical Notes About Cheryl

The following section contains my clinical notes about Cheryl and her progress.

Chief Complaint: Cheryl, a 39-year-old white female, complained of coughing up blood. In July 1996 she was diagnosed with non–small-cell adenocarcinoma of the lung. Before visiting my office, Cheryl had chemotherapy without any response. She came to me for a second opinion.

Diagnostics: Chest x-ray, bronchoscopy, thoracotomy, EDS (electrodermal screening), BTA (biological terrain assessment), food allergy tests, hair mineral analysis, comprehensive hormone profile

Physical Exam: Normal except for four silver fillings (amalgams)

Results: Tests for mercury indicated high mercury toxicity and arsenic.

Treatments: Chelation therapy, detoxification, coffee enema, juicing, gallbladder-liver flush, Sanum homeopathic remedies

Commentary: Mercury is received from many sources including silver fillings, air pollution, sea food, cosmetics, and vaccinations. Silver fillings are commonly composed of approximately 50% mercury, 20% silver, 20% copper, and 10% tin. The percentages vary depending on the specific amalgam.

Treatment: Mercury is one of the most neurotoxic substances that has been commonly used in dentistry and has escaped into our environment as an industrial waste. Therefore, the first step of detoxification was to give Cheryl a series of chelation treatments using DMPS to help her body remove the mercury. Cheryl also had all her amalgams replaced with nonmetal composites.

What is DMPS?

DMPS is an abbreviation for dimercaptopropane sulfonate that is used for chelation therapy. Chelation therapy, performed on an outpatient basis at a doctor's office, is a safe and effective treatment for heavy-metal toxicity. It is effective for many illnesses because free radicals and inflammation, caused by heavy metals, are neutralized when the heavy metals are bound and extracted from the contaminated tissues and organs.

There are many standard pharmaceutical-chelating agents available for heavy-metal toxicity in both oral and intravenous form that are available through the care of a physician. DMPS is a chelating agent that has been used for mercury and lead toxicity in Europe for over 50 years.

DMPS is an example of a chelating agent that is administered intravenously. My intravenous infusion room is filled with lounge chairs where patients relax while they wait for the chelating agent to drip intravenously.

Support therapy to aid in cleansing and detoxification included *Chlorella*, chlorophyll, glutathione, a combination of antioxidants, vitamins and minerals, and Sanum homeopathic remedies. Cheryl also had a daily coffee enema, organic carrot and green vegetable juices, and a monthly gallbladder-liver flush.

Outcome: Cheryl's mercury level dramatically dropped. Within 6 months of starting the treatment programs, all of Cheryl's tumor disappeared. A CT scan showed only scar tissue in her lungs.

Cheryl continues on a maintenance dose of DMPS chelation once a month, coffee enema a couple times weekly, juicing a couple times weekly, and a gallbladder-liver flush quarterly.

Summary: Cheryl, who was supposed to live only 1 year, now reports that her oncology nurse asks her what she does to look so good. At the time of this writing, she has been cancer free for 12 years.

Heavy-metal toxicity is one of the major underlying factors in weakening the immune system and has to be addressed for all cancer patients.

Success Story: Stage 4 Cancer Gone and Chemo Tolerance "Easier"

The following note is from a patient whose thymoma (cancer of the thymus) cancer disappeared after treatment:

Dear Dr. Yu and Staff,

On February 14, 2007 I received some incredible news about my health. As a 45-year-old man, diagnosed with Stage 4 cancer in August of 2005, a recent PET scan revealed that all remaining cancer from surgery was nonexistent. The care I received from you and your staff beginning in September 2005 was outstanding. It helped me get through three tough rounds of chemotherapy by getting me back on my feet much quicker than anticipated.

After undergoing the first round of chemotherapy without being under your care, I can certainly attest to the fact that the next three seemed much easier to contend with. Your care gave me hope. It pulled me through a very difficult time, and now you have made my body strong once again.

I will now turn to you for prevention, to keep any recurrence from happening. I have been and will continue spreading the good news about you, your treatments, and wonderful staff. Your approach to health needs to be recognized.

> *My sincerest thanks,*
> *K. F.*

Success Story: Kidney Cancer Follow-Up and Immune Building

This patient has provided readers with a great deal of detail about his experience with kidney cancer.

From one day to the next, I developed kidney cancer! Of course, it wasn't in just one day. It had been developing for some time. How long, no one will ever know. Very fast in one month? Slowly over several years? Or some time in between? I went in the hospital at 9:00 AM one morning and by 5:00 PM I'm going into surgery to have my right kidney removed…and the tumor was half the size of the kidney. I was "fortunate," not, of course, in having the cancer, but in that the cancer had not spread outside my kidney. Therefore, I did not have any follow-up chemotherapy or radiation.

After the initial shock and scare of having cancer and recovering from the surgery, the next step was to have follow-up exams. Even though I had utilized homeopathy, which is one aspect of alternative medicine, I was so scared by the thought of cancer and the words from the conventional medical establishment that I went to a nationally renowned hospital for follow-up. I was on the "fringe" of alternative medicine, not having fully embraced it because I simply knew too little about it. My follow-up consisted of x-rays and blood work every 6 months, and CAT scans once a year.

I kept wondering what they—the medical professionals—and I were doing with this information. It finally dawned on me that all they were doing was waiting, waiting to see when cancer would return. They were checking to see if they could catch it in its early stages, as if they could treat it any better by catching it early. After all, the cancer studies follow patients for 5 years, as if that's enough to extend one's life. After over 30 years and over $35 billion spent on cancer research, cancer rates are still increasing. Doesn't this suggest that maybe this research is looking in the wrong places to cure it? How about the novel idea of just taking all of the known carcinogens out of our environment and eliminating toxic products and manufacturing processes so people don't get cancer in the first place? But, I digress.

I started my own serious research and reading into alternative medicine for cancer. A "lightbulb" finally lit up in my head one day when logic and common sense took hold of me. My thinking went like this: I realized that everyone has cancerous cells. A healthy immune system keeps them in check; kills them off. Since I got cancer, my immune system must have broken down. Therefore, why don't I remove all the causes of cancer for which I have control and also build the strength of my immune system? Yes, that's exactly what I decided to do.

In my research, I developed a three-point plan. First, I learned of many diagnostic tests that conventional medicine was not using that provided much better and more complete information about the health of my entire body and all its or-

gans. I made a list of all the tests that I wanted to have done. Second, I made a list of preventive actions that I wanted to take, including a variety of nutritional support. Third, I made a list of alternative medicine therapies that I would use if cancer should return.

I ran into a friend of mine who told me how Dr. Yu had helped his wife get her health back after conventional doctors had "messed her up" with all the prescription drugs and their side effects and interactions. I was amazed when I first took my lists into Dr. Yu and found that he was using all the diagnostic tests and preventive treatments on my lists plus many more that I hadn't considered. He was using a variety of therapies that drew upon the best that alternative medicine and conventional medicine have to offer. I had found the hope and active health guide I was seeking.

When I started with Dr. Yu, I began my "second half" of recovering from cancer. Most conventional medical professionals exclusively focus on ridding the body of cancer. They destroy the body and its immune system while attempting to kill the cancer with the poison of chemotherapy and by burning it out with radiation. Of the conventional treatments, surgery is the least destructive to the immune system. The cancer, however, may only be "conquered" temporarily. The "other half" of conquering cancer is to make sure it doesn't return.

Since starting with Dr. Yu, we discovered I had mercury toxicity, parasites, and weakened organ functions. In my alternative medicine research, I found that these are a few of the many causes of weakened immune systems that can lead to cancer or a variety of other illnesses. These "weak links" of my body have been remedied through the following actions: replacement of all my mercury fillings (I like to call them what they really are and not the euphemistic name of "silver" fillings), chelation for removal of mercury in my body, para-

site cleansing, and nutritional support to strengthen weak organ function and build my immune system. I continue with periodic monitoring of my "biological terrain." This monitoring determines adjustments in my immune-building routines to keep me on the right track.

There are no guarantees in life. But I feel I am now taking the positive, proactive steps to maximize my chances that cancer will not return so I can live a healthy life. I am extremely thankful that Dr. Yu has chosen to use his knowledge, training, talents, and skills toward what I consider to be the true practice of healing.

E.M.

Success Story: Breast Cancer and Removal of Mercury

This female patient relays her experience with mercury removal after her experience with breast cancer.

I began treatments to remove my mercury fillings in August of 1999. We completed the treatment by December 1999.

I would like to report the improvements in my health:

My energy levels, as well as depression, are much improved. My mental abilities have improved. I have more memory, clarity, and improved cognitive reasoning skills. My level of mercury has decreased from 75 to 17 within 6 months.

In the past 13 months, I have been focused on healing my body and spirit after my treatments from breast cancer.

Removing heavy metals from my body has been one of the main focuses. I also need to interject that changing the acid base part of my body, the chiropractic, along with other modalities have all added to my increasing great health. My energy levels have greatly increased. My depression, fatigue, apathy, and grief have decreased to a point where I no longer identify with those emotions. My hair and skin are outward signs of my increasing healthy body.

If I were to tell "my story" to a group of cancer patients and offer a checklist of essential steps to heal themselves, removing heavy metals (mercury) would be top on the list.

D.C.

Success Story: Tongue Cancer

Here is another story from my clinical notes about a female who had tongue cancer.

Chief Complaint: Karen, an 86-year-old white female from Chicago, IL, came to see me in July 1998 with a history of cancer of the tongue diagnosed in December 1997. She had a partial resection of the tongue and had recurrent squamous cell cancer. Her oncologist recommended radiation therapy. Karen decided to seek a second opinion.

Diagnostics: EDS (electrodermal screening also known as Acupuncture Meridian Assessment), hair mineral analysis

Physical Exam: Normal exam except multiple amalgams and squamous cell tumor at the apex of the tongue

Results: EDS revealed a disturbance to the dental meridian and joint problems. Hair mineral analysis revealed aluminum toxicity.

Treatments: Homeopathic remedies for dental and lymphatic drainage plus *Chlorella* and green chlorophyll. Karen was instructed to remove her amalgams in Chicago.

Treatment: Karen had her silver-mercury amalgams replaced.

Outcome: Karen next visited my office in September 2000 for unrelated problems. During a discussion of her cancer, she told me that, immediately after one-half of her amalgams were removed, the cancer spontaneously disappeared. She reported that her oral surgeon had commented to her that he had never seen this happen. She completed the removal of her amalgams and has been cancer free since December 2001 when I had a conversation with her daughter.

Summary: Usually cancer patients require extensive detoxification and nutritional supplementation to reverse the cancer. Heavy metals have often been one of the cofactors that are strongly associated with cancerous conditions and often require extensive chelation therapy to remove the heavy-metal toxicity. Karen's case was very unusual in that the cancer resolved itself with minimal detoxification.

15

Solving Lung and
Heart Problems

*Every time I came down with bronchitis. I would run to
my local primary care physician who put me on antibiotics.
My health was a roller coaster ride between
ill to fair to ill again.*
S.E. (Patient)

This chapter presents case histories and related testimonials of patients who developed lung and heart problems from underlying factors that I see in nearly all of my patients, regardless of their disease patterns.

Heart disease is still the nation's #1 killer, and lung cancer is the nation's top cancer killer. Both of these diseases have responded to the therapies that I use to restore balance in meridians:

- Nutrition
- Antiparasite herbs, homeopathics and/or prescription drugs
- Dental evaluation and treatment by a biological dentist
- Food allergy tests and an elimination diet
- Chelation
- Liver-gallbladder flush
- Oil pulling

Success Story: Worms Expelled From Bronchial Tubes

This first case study is probably the most dramatic of all of my patient stories. At 38, Valerie leads a busy professional life running a business in Kansas City with her husband. She is also the mother of four children and is very comfortable sharing the details about her experience with worms that she expelled from her body after taking prescription anti-parasite medication. What's most compelling about Valerie's story are her symptoms and the fact that her symptoms disappeared when she expelled what she described as a large fluke and pinworms from her mouth, as well as a tapeworm from her gastrointestinal tract.

Valerie's Neck "Closed" and She Could Not Breathe

At the height of her unexplained physical problems, Valerie says her blocked breathing was frightening, and it's this symptom that brought her to my office. She describes the feeling of her blocked breathing as her "neck closing." Although she had difficulty breathing, her doctors could not find anything physically wrong with her. They thought she had an atypical form of asthma.

Valerie's blocked breathing was just one of her health problems, and all of her symptoms mystified her doctors. She describes one of her

---

Parasites Secrete Toxins and Steal Nutrients

There are over 100 different types of parasite worms that can live in the human body.

Worm Embryos Form Cysts That Infect Animal Flesh
When an undeveloped tapeworm infects an animal host, it can drill through the abdominal lining and get into the bloodstream where arteries and veins become highways. It can then find its way to the liver or a large muscle and form a fluid sac called a cyst. The young tapeworm can live inside a cyst until the animal's flesh is eaten by some other animal.

worst symptoms as "yellow bile peeing out of my butt for almost two years." A colorectal specialist whom she saw for the pain and discomfort convinced her that this problem was related to hemorrhoids, and he performed hemorrhoid surgery. Other problems included double sciatica, uncontrolled facial twitching, panic attacks, and chronic bladder infections. Although the parasite medication has alleviated many of Valerie's symptoms, she still has back pain. Valerie's history, which is explained in this chapter, provides clues that mirror underlying problems faced by most of my patients:

- Chemical and heavy-metal toxins
- Recurring parasite infections due to a polluted terrain

Doctors Do Not Look for Worms

Parasites are so hidden in the United States that only a handful of doctors look for them. As we will see as we cover her case, Valerie's parasites were able to invade her body because of her weakened

---

Treating Patients Who Live Far Away

Valerie is an example of a patient who lives in a city that is several hours from my clinic. Although I treat many patients who live far away, it is always a challenge—particularly when it comes to treating parasite infections.

A weakened immune system has trouble fighting parasites on its own, and I often need to prescribe several rounds of antiparasite medications before a patient's symptoms are resolved. It is hard to say whether Valerie's continued back pain is due to hidden invaders.

immune system. What's important to understand is that all Americans are vulnerable to parasites, and I'm convinced that they are the underlying cause of many health problems. Until they are diagnosed, many people will have a hard time recovering from their illnesses.

Traumas Often Push the Immune System Into a State of Imbalance

In many cases, a patient's trauma can push an already compromised immune system into a state of imbalance. Valerie traces her breathing problem to an accident on a lake where she and her husband have a summer home. She fell off a dock and swallowed a lot of lake water and had trouble breathing the next day. While it's possible that the lake water was the source of her parasite infection, her immune system was already compromised when she fell off the dock, and the incident may have accelerated her decline.

Parasites Rob Us of Our Life Force

A parasite infection is extremely debilitating. Parasites live off our life force and the food that we eat. In addition to a resultant loss of nutrition and cellular damage, the toxins produced by parasites play havoc with our immune system. An infection can mimic other diseases, such as irritable bowel, chronic fatigue, Crohn's disease, fibromyalgia, joint pain, and depression.

Parasites are highly intelligent in their ability to survive and reproduce. They can hide in body tissues and avoid detection for many years.

The pH Scale

Acids are defined as those solutions that have a pH less than 7 (or more hydrogen ions than water); while bases are defined as those solutions that have a pH greater than 7 (or less hydrogen ions than water).

Patient Stories Illustrate Concepts and Ideas That May Be New To Readers

This patient story, as well as others in this book, help to illustrate several concepts and ideas that may be new to readers including:

- **Biological Terrain**
  Biological terrain is the biochemical environment of the body that includes the blood, urine, and saliva. The health of the biological terrain can be determined with pH measurements reflecting the acidity or alkalinity of body fluids. pH is an acronym for "potential hydrogen" and refers to the concentration of hydrogen ions (See: The pH Scale).

- **Meridians**
  Meridians are subtle flow of energy in the body that were discovered in China several thousand years ago. The Chinese named 12 principal meridians for the life functions associated with them.

- **Acupuncture Meridian Assessment (AMA)**
  Acupuncture Meridian Assessment (AMA) is the measurement of energy flow through the meridians of the body using an electroacupuncture according to Voll (EAV) device.

- **Therapies That Rebalance Meridians**
  Nutrition and detoxification are the underlying keys to staying healthy.

- **Measures Required to Stay Healthy in Today's Toxic World**
  Detoxification has become an important preventive strategy to enable the body to cope with pollution. Realistically, detox has become an important strategy to stay healthy. Once a patient has rebalanced his/her meridians, the following measures are recommended as maintenance measures:

    - *Liver-gallbladder flush (every quarter)*
    - *Oil pulling (daily)*
    - *Maintenance dose of antiparasite herbs (biannually)*

Valerie's Meridian Imbalances

Valerie's parasites were detected with an electroacupuncture according to Voll (EAV) device that I use to measure the electrical voltage at 54 acupuncture points on a patient's hands and feet. A patient whose health has declined may have as many as 50 readings that show a meridian imbalance. Healthy patients can have as many as 7 to 10 imbalances and show no symptoms of disease.

As I explain in other chapters in this book, the evaluation tool that I use is a meridian-based technology that was developed by a German scientist and physician named Dr. Reinhard Voll. Voll's technology uses electrical "norms" or baseline electrical voltages reflecting the energy levels of meridian-associated organs.

One of the main reasons that parasites go undiagnosed is because parasitology labs fail to find the majority of intestinal parasites in stool specimens submitted to them. For example, the test of a routine stool evaluation for ova and parasites picks up less than 10 percent of active infections.

The Voll machine's metal platform provides a means to match the energetic frequency of a parasite infection and a remedy. When a medication is placed on the platform, it becomes part of the body's electrical circuit, and the changes that occur in an acupoint reading provide a clue that a patient has parasites. If a medication that is placed on the machine's metal platform produces a positive change in a meridian, it is also a valuable clue that the medication will kill the parasite.

Hair Analysis Provides Details About Essential and Toxic Minerals

Hair analysis is a valuable diagnostic tool that has been used by alternative doctors for several decades. The test provides helpful clues about the ratios of essential minerals that we need for our metabolism, as well as toxic mineral levels. Valerie's test showed mercury and aluminum. Of these, mercury is the most serious and may be due to her two root canals and a crown.

Root Canals and Crowns Often Contain Mercury

Although dental amalgam is the largest source of mercury, some root canals are filled with mercury, and crowned teeth often have mercury underneath. When dentists grind a tooth for a crown, they often leave a mercury-filled stub if the tooth had a filling. Valerie mentioned that her dentist recently replaced her root canals and said he found an infection in her jaw that he guessed was there for 18 years. Valerie also mentioned that she developed dry sockets after her wisdom teeth were removed. Mercury, root-canaled teeth, and cavitations are common causes of chronic health problems such as chronic fatigue, fibromyalgia, multiple sclerosis, as well as many other health problems. Valerie will not truly stay healthy until all her dental work is completed.

Success Story: Bronchial Symptoms Resolved in Three Months

This section contains a letter from a male patient who struggled with bronchitis for 3 years.

Dear Dr. Yu:

I have been a relatively healthy person until about 3 years ago when I came down with recurring bronchitis and pneumonia from which I was unable to fully recover. Soon after I was diagnosed with bronchiectasis, a condition where the lungs don't work properly to rid mucus from the airways, making any type of physical activity (this includes walking) demanding and exhausting. Another consequence of this condition is mucus remains in the lungs and serves as an ideal environment for bacteria colonization, hence the frequent bouts of bronchitis and pneumonia I experienced over the years since.

I'm thankful that doctors at Washington University's Center for Advanced Medicine were able to stabilize my symptoms through medications, inhalers, a nebulizer machine, and antibiotic therapy as needed. As it turned out, this protocol was simply managing my symptoms and treating my lung infections as they occurred, which were five to six times a year for the past 2 years.

Every time I came down with bronchitis, I would run to my local primary care physician who put me on antibiotics of some variety. If my condition didn't improve in a few days, I would call the doctors at Washington University and let them have a look and see what other medicines/therapy might be needed. My heath was a roller-coaster ride between ill to fair to ill again.

Doctors advised me that this was the scenario I could expect for the rest of my life, but that I could lead a relatively normal life. The relatively normal part of this explanation bothered me tremendously.

It was hard to accept this as a way of life for a 43-year-old person, since I had enjoyed robust, if not exceptional, health nearly all of my life up to this point.

For starters, I wasn't a smoker and rarely drank alcohol but on special occasions, and rarely to excess. I was also fairly prudent about my diet, avoiding junk foods and empty calorie foodstuffs. I take vitamins and supplements daily, and exercise regularly. So this diagnosis came as a complete surprise, but surprising further was that nobody seemed interested in finding a possible "cause."

The first year I started experiencing these symptoms, I missed 40 days of work and probably should have missed more. The second year I missed 20 days of work—a 100% improvement, but a far cry from what I considered normal.

Throughout this time, I had conversations with many people about health and wellness options and opinions. One notable conversation was with a woman with whom I work named Nancy. She informed me that a friend of hers was going to see a doctor, an M.D., who used both conventional and alternative therapies, as traditional doctors had been unable to help her. I can't recall exactly what her symptoms were, but she wanted another opinion. To make a long story short, the doctor the woman was going to see was Dr. Yu. Without much hesitation, I decided to set up an appointment, since I felt as if I was in the same boat. Besides, what did I have to lose, anyway?

Well, I must admit my first visit with Dr. Yu was bewildering. I was analyzed with some odd-looking (and sounding) medical equipment, the likes of which I had never seen in my other doctors' offices. Nevertheless, I remained open minded and agreed to at least give this stuff a try. Some of the equipment I recall having read about in alternative medicine books and newsletters to which I subscribe.

Actually seeing the machines in action with my body as the test sub-ject was intriguing, to say the least. One particular machine, the Acupuncture Meridian Assessment, tested various acupuncture points on the hands and feet and was able to identify abnormal tissues/organs using an electrical impulse. My test revealed abnormalities in the lower intestines and lungs and a few other readings were low, which is considered to be abnormal.

In relation to these readings, Dr. Yu was fairly certain, but not posi-tive, that I might have a parasite infection. Although the notion that I could be infested with parasites was unnerving, I agreed to submit to a regimen of supplements and prescription medication, thinking what did I have to lose but a little bit of money (and parasites!) in the big picture. My health was certainly worth giving it a try, and if I didn't try it, I'd never know whether it might help.

Dr. Yu explained to me that during the treatment to eradicate para-sites I might have a flare-up of my symptoms, but not to be alarmed as this would pass in a few days. Well, sure enough after the first month or so of treatment, I came down with what I thought was another bout of bronchitis—fever and coughing up mucus.

Having been so dependent on conventional treatment and not want-ing my symptoms to progress into anything worse, I panicked and called my primary care doctor, and he put me on antibiotics, as usual. I figured I should at least let Dr. Yu know about my condition to see if there would be any contraindications in combining the anti-biotics and the parasite treatment.

Well, right away he wanted to see me in his office. He explained that my symptoms were a normal and expected process of the parasite cycle, in that the parasites were dying out. He insisted that I didn't need antibiotics and showed me, using the Acupuncture Meridian Assessment machine, how the antibiotic I was taking wouldn't help.

I had a hard time with the notion that I didn't need antibiotics when I felt this ill, but I was willing to take his advice. To fight the infection that was being caused by the parasites dying off, Dr. Yu recommended that I take 2000 mg of Vitamin C every hour until I reached bowel intolerance (diarrhea), and then reduce the dosage when this normalized. I went home and began taking Vitamin C as prescribed and in less than 5 hours (after taking a total of 10,000 mg of Vitamin C), my fever broke and I was beginning to feel better. Every day thereafter I felt a little bit better.

It's been nearly 5 months since I first visited Dr. Yu, and I can tell you that I haven't felt this good in over 3 years. During my last 2 appointments, the Acupuncture Meridian Assessment indicated all my meridians were in the normal range. My strength and stamina have returned and my improvements amaze me.

I work out nearly every day and can now perform over 20 pull-ups and 50 push-ups—feats I could only dream of accomplishing less than 3 years ago. I have gained back nearly 20 lbs of muscle and just recently went rock climbing in Wyoming, keeping up with my wife (11 years my junior) and my niece and her boyfriend, both in their early 20s. Although my lung function will probably never be normal due to scarring and past infections, I can do all the things I ever hoped of doing. And now all of this prescription drug free!

Thank you, Dr. Yu, for giving me a new and improved lease on life.

> *Sincerely,*
> *S.E.*

Success Story: Bronchial Symptoms and Numerous Other Problems

This section contains a report from a female patient who struggled with bronchitis, anxiety, depression, allergies from jewelry, and poor night vision.

For the first time in my life, I can honestly say that, after undergoing extensive dental treatment, I am feeling well. Prior to seeing Dr. Rehme (dentist), I had gone through two regimens of dental treatment at two area dental schools. After the first, I was diagnosed with severe depression and began to suffer recurrent bouts of bronchitis. After the second, I developed acute anxiety and paranoia, a sclerosis of the cornea (shadow vision), which made it impossible to do any extensive reading, contact dermatitis (which prevented me from wearing jewelry), and severe pet allergies.

One year ago, I found that I was suffering from acute mercury toxicity. Several upper molars had shattered around their mercury amalgams. The mercury amalgams were removed from my lower molars and replaced with porcelain. The mercury amalgams in two other teeth were replaced with nontoxic materials. My mercury levels were reduced with DMPS IVs (intravenous injections) to a level where I can now take DMSA orally. I am continuing to take vitamin and mineral supplements and am still doing periodic liver-gallbladder flushes.

Since beginning treatment with Drs. Yu and Rehme, I have not had a single bout of bronchitis. I no longer suffer anxiety or depression. I am able to wear jewelry without breaking out and not only has my shadow vision improved to the point that I can now safely drive at night, but I can even sometimes read without my glasses—for the first time since the 6th grade!

My pet allergies are even a little better. My students no longer complain about my illegible handwriting. We are about halfway through the treatment program. I am very optimistic about my full recovery.

The AMA- and ADA-approved treatments I received almost ruined my health and my life.

B.A.

Success Story: Asthma and Multiple Other Mysterious Problems

This patient saw numerous doctors who kept coming up with new diagnoses.

Dr. Yu and Staff,

Here is a testimonial I have written and would be more than willing to share with other patients hopefully to encourage. I am so thankful for everything you have done and continue to do for me!

About 4 years ago, I became very ill and began having strange symptoms, such as nosebleeds, difficulty breathing, dizziness, fatigue, headaches, lymph node swelling, and pain throughout my body. I was exposed to a high amount of toxic mold, which has been the cause of what I believe to be the majority of these symptoms.

My immune system really took a dip, and I developed mononucleosis. I was sent to numerous doctors, most diagnosing me with asthma, chronic fatigue, and sinusitis directly from the mold. Scariest of all, I was diagnosed with demyelination of the central nervous system due to what the doctors think to be a prolonged suppressed immune system.

I had several tests, including an eye test, hearing test, CT scans, and MRIs, that revealed this to be the issue. I was having tingling in my arms and legs, headaches, pains in sides/back, leg pain, feet/ toe twitching, eye twitching, dizziness, extreme fatigue, a hard time sleeping, gastrointestinal issues, and much more.

There were approximately 3-4 spots found on my brain, and the doctor wanted to do a spinal tap to rule out MS. This is not mention-ing the numerous specialists I saw prior to this treatment, and they just couldn't seem to find what was wrong. I followed different types of treatment along with a strict organic and natural diet (I still do try to eat healthy).

I even flew and drove to Texas a couple times to see a toxicologist who did some fungal treatment for the mold issue, and blood work that cost a fortune. I still had no answers.

Needless to say, I was extremely frustrated, discouraged, and had no money left!!! I looked up a doctor's name who happened to live in Illinois, and who had helped people like myself, hoping maybe this would finally be the right answer. He actually said, "Oh, you're from Missouri? There is a doctor right there in St. Louis that could probably help you."

He gave me Dr. Yu's name and contact information. That was what I needed to hear. I still felt it was just too good to be true. I saw Dr. Yu and he did an exam, and also Acupuncture Meridian Assessment. The Acupuncture Meridian Assessment revealed several problems that were affecting me and possibly causing the very problems I was experiencing.

Dr. Yu treated me for several issues to improve my health. My husband, family, friends, and coworkers were amazed at how I was recovering. I continue to be treated by Dr. Yu today (8 months later). I feel so much better, and I am finally feeling normal again. I have energy and can work out (not as much as I would like, but gaining every day that passes).

It is such a wonderful thing just to feel good. My last monthly evaluation revealed that nothing else has appeared, and the neurologist said he would just monitor it now with MRIs.

My last visit with Dr. Yu was extremely encouraging as he reported to me that my Acupuncture Meridian Assessment was normal, and my body seemed to be doing well. I know it is because I feel it!!! I thank the good Lord for healing me because I know he has. I also thank the Lord because I truly feel he led me to Dr. Yu at Prevention and Healing.

That is truly what Dr. Yu's practice is about, preventing and healing! Dr. Yu's office staff are remarkable. They are so kind, compassionate, and always willing to lend a hand or help in any way possible.

I cannot think of another doctor under whose care I would prefer to be than Dr. Yu. His care for me has been unbelievable!

I am a teacher, and it takes a great amount of energy to fulfill that job. I am able to really enjoy my job now. I have referred several of my friends and family members who have issues that their doctors cannot seem to figure out. I know there are good doctors out there, but I truly believe Dr. Yu is the best.

God Bless,

M.A.

Success Story: Scleroderma Stabilized

The following section contains my clinical notes about a female with scleroderma, a connective tissue disease that can affect the skin, blood vessels, muscles, and internal organs. Conventional medicine has no treatment for scleroderma, and the disease can be fatal. Two thirds of patients with scleroderma have respiratory problems, such as shortness of breath, coughing, and difficulty breathing.

Chief Complaint: Barb, a 55-year-old female, was diagnosed with scleroderma. She had restrictive lung problems and fatigue symptoms —typical in patients with scleroderma.

Diagnostics: EDS (electrodermal screening), hair mineral analysis, DMPS chelation challenge test for heavy-metal toxicity

Physical Exam: Barb had approximately 15 amalgams. Her fingers were swollen like sausages, which severely limited her range of motion.

Results: EDS revealed lymph drainage problems, liver and stomach disturbances, and kidney and gallbladder disturbances. Hair analysis revealed excessive calcium and aluminum levels. The DMPS chelation challenge test indicated Barb had a very high mercury toxicity level.

Treatments: I recommended having all her amalgams replaced, as well as chelation therapy to remove the heavy metals along with nutritional supplementation.

Commentary: The cause of scleroderma was initially unknown. Barb did not act on my recommendation to replace her amalgams for about a year. Then one day one of her amalgams just fell out, and she immediately noticed that she could move one of her fingers much more freely than previously. She then decided to have all her amalgams replaced.

Outcome: After having all of Barb's amalgams replaced, she had additional improvement in her finger joint movement. Barb's restrictive lung disease has improved as indicated by a pulmonary function test. Her scleroderma has been stabilized.

Summary: Proper dental treatment and heavy-metal detoxification is indicated for all autoimmune disorders of unknown cause.

Success Story: Atrial Fibrillation and Congestive Heart Failure

The following section contains my clinical notes about a female who had an abnormal heart rhythm known as atrial fibrillation (AF) and congestive heart failure (CHF). CHF is a condition in which the heart has trouble pumping blood to the other organs of the body.

Chief Complaint: Judy, an 87-year-old female, came to see me in September 1995, complaining of atrial fibrillation and congestive heart failure. Her cardiac ejection fraction was 21%. (Her heart can only pump at 21% efficiency compared to a normal 65%.) The prognosis she was previously given for her condition was approximately one year to live at most.

Diagnostics: Hair mineral analysis, food allergy tests, blood tests

Physical Exam: Judy's irregular heartbeat was consistent with atrial fibrillation. Judy has been on multiple medications without any sign of edema (swelling).

Results: Hair mineral analysis did not indicate anything exceptional. Food allergy tests indicated multiple allergies to dairy products, eggs, papaya, almonds, lima beans, sesame, green pepper, and squash.

Treatments: Judy had intravenous EDTA chelation treatments at one per week for 30 treatments. She took coenzyme Q10, L-carnitine, hawthorn berries, cayenne pepper, melatonin, vitamins and minerals based on the hair mineral analysis results, intravenous vitamins and minerals once per week for 10 treatments, and coffee enemas.

Commentary: Congestive heart failure with an ejection fraction at 21% is literally a "death sentence" especially at an advanced age.

Outcome: Judy's ejection fraction increased to 35%. Judy's treatment added 10 years to her life. She died at age 97.

Summary: Judy was very open minded about alternative medicine and actively pursued my recommendations. Her attitude and persistence in following a prescribed course of action paid off considerably for her.

Success Story: Coronary Artery Disease (Bypass Surgery Avoided)

The following section contains my clinical notes about a female with coronary artery disease, which is an accumulation of plaque on the walls of the coronary arteries. The photograph on the following page is an image of a coronary artery taken through a microscope showing a narrowing called atherosclerosis.

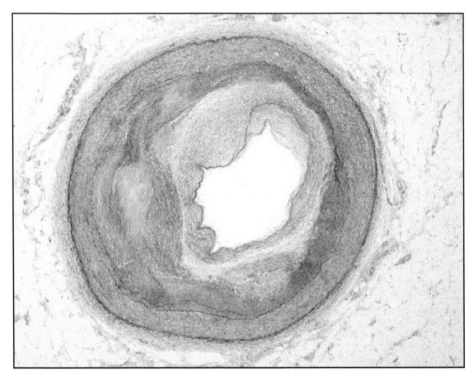

Photo: Image of a coronary artery taken through a microscope showing a narrowing called atherosclerosis.

Chief Complaint: Jane, a 55-year-old female, complained of chest pain. She had a history of juvenile diabetes, diabetic neuropathy, and diabetic retinopathy. Her heart specialist recommended a triple bypass operation. She decided to seek alternatives to a bypass procedure.

Diagnostics: Angiogram, EDS (electrodermal screening), hair mineral analysis

Physical Exam: Normal exam except 8 silver fillings (amalgams) and decreased sensation in the lower extremities from the diabetic neuropathy

Results: Tests for mercury indicated extremely high mercury toxicity.

Commentary: Mercury is received from many sources including silver fillings, air pollution, seafood, cosmetics, and vaccinations. Silver fillings are commonly composed of approximately 50% mercury, 20% silver, 20% copper, 10% tin. The percentages vary depending on the specific amalgam.

Treatments: Chelation therapy, detoxification, and nutritional therapy. Jane also had all her amalgams replaced with nonmetal composites.

Mercury is one of the most neurotoxic substances that has been commonly used in dentistry and has escaped into our environment as an industrial waste. Therefore, the first step of detoxification was to give Jane a series of chelation treatments using DMPS to help her body remove the mercury. She was then given an oral chelation agent, DMSA, and started on EDTA chelation.

Support therapy to aid in cleansing and detoxification included *Chlorella*, chlorophyll, glutathione, and a combination of antioxidants, vitamins, and minerals.

Outcome: Jane's mercury level dramatically dropped to near-normal levels. Her clinical symptoms of angina have disappeared. She reported that she went to Europe and accomplished a lot of climbing of hills without any chest pain.

Jane continues on a maintenance dose of EDTA chelation once a month and follows the peak-performance diet that I recommended.

Summary: Jane avoided a bypass operation, which would have addressed only a symptom of her condition. By eliminating the heavy-metal toxicity of mercury, providing nutritional support, and controlling free radical damage, the causes of her chest pain were addressed.

Success Story: Idiopathic Thrombocytopenic Purpura (ITP)

The following section contains my clinical notes about a 3-year-old boy with low blood platelet counts disorder, otherwise known as idiopathic thrombocytopenic purpura (ITP). About 50 to 100 cases (per million people in the population) of ITP show up each year and half are children.

Chief Complaint: Joey, a 3-year-old boy, came to see me with a diagnosis of ITP at age 2. He had a platelet count of 10,000 compared to a typical average of 250,000. He had been on steroids without response. Joey's hematologist recommended removal of the spleen to treat the ITP. His initial symptom was that he bruised easily.

Diagnostics: Blood test for platelet counts, EDS (electrodermal screening), food allergy tests, hair mineral analysis

Physical Exam: Normal

Results: Lead and aluminum toxicity indicated by hair mineral analysis; food allergies indicated, including cow's milk, wheat, soy, corn, buckwheat, yogurt, and many others.

Treatments: Parasite cleansing therapy, homeopathic chelation therapy, food rotation diet, and antifungal remedies

Outcome: Joey came to see me a total of 4 times. His platelet count increased from 10,000 to 250,000 in a period of 1 year. According to Joey's mother, he has been doing very well. He is very active and does not bruise easily any more. Joey and his parents happily avoided a spleenectomy.

Summary: Joey's mother told the hematologist about Joey's progress. The hematologist said he was not interested in what I did, but that it was possible Joey never had ITP. If this were true, the hematologist obviously would have recommended a totally unnecessary operation.

16

Leaky Gut, Leaky Brain
Irritable Bowel, Irritable Mind

Twenty years of symptoms and pain
disappeared in eleven months.
Colonel H. (Patient)

Patients with gastrointestinal complaints often have a myriad of other health problems due to compromised immune systems. The human immune system is very much dependent on a healthy gastrointestinal tract.

While the case histories in this chapter may also include other symptoms, gastrointestinal distress was a primary factor that led them to my clinic.

Success Story: Twenty Years of Symptoms Gone in Eleven Months

This first case study is an insightful story about a patient who lived with several painful symptoms for years. Like so many other patients, this male patient—a Colonel in the Army—struggled with parasites. What struck me the most was his ability to function in the military in spite of his symptoms. His story is also described in my article titled "Operation Enduring Freedom: Saving Colonel H" that has been added to Chapter 6.

Preface (February/Dr. Yu): As I have mentioned in my article in Chapter 6 and elsewhere in the book, I was in the U.S. Army Reserves for 25 years and first saw Colonel H. when I was stationed

at a U.S. Army base in Germany. I detected a major problem with
parasites in Colonel H. Parasites are very common, even in the
developed world and industrialized countries with clean water and
sanitary conditions. What is pertinent to this story and many other
patient stories is the fact that several months are often needed to
treat parasites. I use a variety of more than 20 different natural and
prescription parasite remedies that need to be matched to a person's
individual evaluation. Parasite remedies are often used in a sequence
that combines types of remedies and dosages. Over the years, I have
seen an amazing array of illnesses respond positively to antiparasite
remedies.

When I first saw Colonel H., he also had major dental problems.
Due to his circumstances in the Army, his dental work had to wait to
be addressed.

I returned to the U.S. at the end of March, a month after I first saw
Colonel H. Colonel H.'s treatments needed to continue, and the
solution was to stay in communication and provide guidance while
Colonel H. worked with local Army physicians.

The rest of the comments below are from Colonel H.'s e-mail
messages to me, written over 11 months. As he explains,
Colonel H. had been suffering with a variety of ailments and pain
for 20 years. These problems disappeared in eleven months.

(March/Colonel H.)
*I am so grateful. I will tell you the drugs I take, old symptoms, things
that improved, symptoms in the last 24 hours, and questions on the
challenges ahead.*

Drugs I am taking:

- *Allopurinol for gout. My uric acid level is now down to 6.7*
- *Lisinopril for high blood pressure*

- *Hydrocholorothiazide for high blood pressure*
- *Loratadine for allergies*
- *Indomethacin (one a day for gout prevention)*

Things I suffered from prior to your treatment:

- *High blood pressure (usually 140/90) even with the blood pressure medicine*
- *Bowel problems after eating (feeling bloated, flatulent, and often having diarrhea). Could hear a lot of bowel activity. Problems with my stool.*
- *Fatigue. At the end of the day I just laid on the couch and watched TV.*
- *High feelings of anxiety and anxiousness. I couldn't do things like take time to read or do a jigsaw puzzle. I also could not enjoy what I was doing because I was planning what I was doing next.*
- *Back pain. I had a broken back and arthritis and had pain every day. Was seeing a physical therapist.*
- *Insomnia. I took up to 3 sleeping pills a night and usually at least 1 1/2. Took one at bedtime. I tossed and turned all night and usually had to get up and watch TV between 1-3 AM and take a half sleeping pill.*
- *I have a lot of dental work.*
- *I had previously been treated for amoebic dysentery and Giardia.*
- *Had a headache almost every morning.*
- *Allergies. Had high drainage in the morning and would gag on phlegm. Would gag to the point that in the morning I would throw up a little about 1/3 to 1/4 of the time.*

- *On an EKG in January, I was identified as having an irregular heartbeat in an emergency room while being treated for gout/ bowel problems and shock due to taking high dosages of percocet without a stool softener.*
- *Pretty irritable and on edge all the time.*
- *Always forgetting little stuff like where my keys are located, etc.*
- *At the end of work every day, I would have a desire for alcohol, and at the end of the day, a desire for sleeping pills. Anything to numb myself.*

Behavioral changes (after treatments from me)

- *I liked jigsaw puzzles. Came home and just spent time with my wife as she makes dinner.*
- *In a high-stress job, I was much calmer and approached problem solving differently.*
- *Blood pressure was now 114/77.*
- *Allergies were a lot less. Had to clear my throat a lot, did not have the drainage problems like I had before.*
- *No back pain.*
- *Memory improved. Stopped misplacing items and had better control of my life. Understood complex problems better and easier.*
- *I had no bowel problems. Ate fine and had no flatulence.*
- *No headache. No pain at all.*
- *Slept great. Still used sleeping pills, but usually just one. I woke for a few minutes, got up and used the bathroom, and then went back to sleep. I dreamed, and they were good dreams.*
- *Sex was calmer and more fun with my wife.*
- *No desire for alcohol.*

- *Had much more energy and was more "chatty." Less confrontational and much more cooperative.*
- *Stopped pacing completely.*
- *Changed my plans for the future.*

(Colonel H. ran out of the medications and the treatments needed to be continued as evidenced by the following:

Big changes in the last 24 hours, and I could feel it inside before I noticed physical symptoms.

- *Allergies have increased, and I have noticed a lot of phlegm. I have begun gagging on the phlegm again.*
- *Feelings of anxiousness or anxiety that I can feel around my solar plexus area and below.*
- *Hear much more bowel activity.*
- *Have a little sensation in my stomach after I eat.*
- *More trouble sleeping. Woke up between 1-3 AM and couldn't go back to sleep. Took Zolpidem, and watched TV for a while, then went back to sleep.*
- *Feel under more stress, even though in the past 3 weeks I was under more stress than this week.*
- *Don't have the same feeling of contentment, joy, and calmness. I have remained calmer, but it is more forced rather than naturally occurring as it was 48 hours ago.*
- *Flatulence has increased.*
- *There is pain between my shoulders and lower back.*
- *Started pacing again.*

Way ahead: Advise me if you think I should share this information with my family care physician. I have known him a few years, and I think he was receptive to what you did. He was definitely impressed with the results. I saw him on March 3rd. If you want to prescribe things or need tests run in the context of conventional Army medicine, I think he would be supportive. I defer to you. You know both sides. If I have to pay this out of my pocket, I will. You have truly changed my life, and I am grateful beyond words. It has had a tremendous impact on my family and changed my plans for the future. I thought I was just aging prematurely.

(July/Colonel H.)

Just wanted to thank you again for all you have done. Your treatment has truly changed my life. I am pain free, and my blood pressure is terrific. Your treatment of my parasites, despite all the challenges from the conventional Army medical community, has incredibly improved my quality of life and ability to do my mission. Everybody notices the difference.

(September/Colonel H.)

Thought you would be interested in the latest development. A little more than a week ago the feeling in my gut returned—and the anxiety. So I took the (medicine) that I had in stock. The feeling in my gut and the anxiety left by the second day.

Yesterday I had blood in my urine. So they did a urinalysis, blood labs, and x-rays. Today they did a CAT scan and discovered I have kidney stones, lots of them. Since I don't have any real pain pertaining to that problem (I do have back and neck pain), they told me to monitor and if my pain worsens, to go to the doctor. Overall my health is still greatly improved. This is the only health issue, other than my back hurting, which is also better, since you first treated me in February.

(December/Colonel H.)

I slept without sleeping pills for the first time in 5 years. I again attribute this to your work.

Colonel H.

Success Story: Taste of Metal in the Mouth Disappears

This patient complained of a metal taste in her mouth. Over time, all metals corrode. As metal fillings wear down, the taste of metal becomes more prevalent. Leaching mercury can also be swallowed and can lead to digestive problems. Fortunately, this patient made a commitment to have her mercury removed, and her report describes her progress.

Prior to getting rid of the greatest mercury problems (upper and lower right teeth), I was getting sluggish by 3-4 PM. I have always been known for my limitless energy and never felt "tired" during the day until the last several years.

Further, I had trouble sleeping when I did go to bed, regardless of the time. And there was a "taste" of metal in my mouth.

After the initial replacement, my energy level increased dramatically. There is now no metallic taste at all, and I am sleeping well, whether I go to bed early or late. I seldom fall asleep during movies or theater performances anymore.

I know I still have a way to go, but I am thrilled with my progress.

P.S. Migraine headaches began about 2 years ago, occurring about 1 or 2 times per month. I have not had one since the filling replacement.

Y.W.

Leaky Gut, Leaky Brain: Mind/Body Connection for Irritable Bowel and Irritable Mind

An article I wrote about the mind/body connection fits into this chapter.

🐦 🐦 🐦

Do you have a problem with concentration, sudden extreme fatigue, irritable mood, chronic vague pain, and a foggy brain as if you have a leaky brain that is ready to shut down? You are not alone! There are millions of people suffering with these symptoms.

These symptoms are considered to be nonspecific. A standard medical diagnostic evaluation usually fails to give the medical doctor a clear picture of the underlying causes. The patient is often told "It's all in your head."

Often, these symptoms manifest from a collection of unrecognized food allergies, hypoglycemia, nutritional deficiency, yeast overgrowth, heavy-metal toxicity, food additive toxins, and hidden parasite infections.

Leaky gut and intestinal dysbiosis have been associated with irritable bowel syndrome and with a whole list of symptoms. Most frequently, the symptoms include abdominal cramps, bloating, gas, diarrhea, constipation, general malaise, and fatigue. These are often associated with brain fog and mood swings.

Yeast and fungal problems have been the suspected culprits of irritable bowel syndrome. Many books have been written on intestinal fungal infections, including *The Yeast Syndrome* by Dr. John Trowbridge, M.D., and

The Yeast Connection by Dr. William G. Crook, M.D. For most people, despite aggressive antifungal medications and a yeast-free diet, symptoms persist.

Most fungal problems are a reflection of environmental problems from overuse of antibiotics and environmental exposure to toxins including heavy-metal toxicity and synthetic chemicals. These toxins adversely disturb the gut flora that directly influence our immune system, alter hormonal balance, and disturb metabolism. They may also create a whole host of unexplained medical complaints.

Overgrowth of yeast in the gut disrupts the integrity of the lining of the intestine and can make patients prone to develop food allergies. Yeast overgrowth also disrupts gut neuropeptide production. The neuropeptide in the gut is the same neuropeptide in your brain. The disruption of the gut neuropeptide creates irritable bowel symptoms that lead to an irritable brain.

Neuropeptides are "information molecules," the basic units of language used by cells throughout an organism to communicate across systems, such as the endocrine, neurological, gastrointestinal, and immune systems. Our gut neuropeptides create molecules of emotion for "gut feeling" and direct communication with the brain. I recommend the book, *Molecules of Emotion,* by Dr. Candace B. Pert, Ph.D..

Tastily packaged processed foods with food additives, such as monosodium glutamate (MSG), are a major reason that gut/brain dysfunction is overlooked. Food additives like MSG are used by industrial food giants to enhance taste and cause food cravings.

Many food additives are "excitotoxins" that overstimulate and eventually kill specific brain cells. Aspartame, which is found in many diet sodas, is an example of a well-known excitotoxin.

Excitotoxins play a major role in a growing number of neurological diseases, including Alzheimer's disease, Parkinson's, multiple sclerosis, amyotrophic lateral sclerosis (ALS), seizures, behavioral and psychiatric disorders, compulsive eating, gross obesity, brain tumors, and sudden death syndrome.

MSG labeling has often been disguised under the name of hydrolyzed proteins, vegetable proteins, soy concentrate or isolates, protein isolates, and natural flavor broth. Please read the important information on excitotoxins by Russell L. Blaylock, M.D., at www.russellblaylockmd.com.

The first line of therapy for leaky gut is to stop using antibiotics for common minor infections, stop eating hormone-fed animal products, and stop eating all forms of sugars, including all grains, alcohol, and fruit juices. Food allergy testing is mandatory for people suffering from what I call a leaky gut/leaky brain syndrome. A common food allergen called gluten also behaves like an excitotoxin in people who are sensitive.

People who have symptoms of a leaky gut should also introduce normal intestinal flora by eating and drinking fermented foods such as yogurt, kefir, buttermilk, sauerkraut, and kimchi. Probiotic supplements, nutritional supplements, and intestinal herbal cleansers are helpful. A gallbladder/liver flush is also a powerful, yet inexpensive method for internal cleansing.

Unrecognized parasite infections are an overlooked factor in patients who have leaky gut symptoms. These infections disrupt the gut lining, making it more susceptible to food allergens and excitotoxins. Most parasites affect areas in the body outside of the gastrointestinal tract as they travel throughout the body. I have written about these parasite destinations many times in articles that may be downloaded from my Web site at www.preventionandhealing.com

In summary, the mind/body connection starts with the quality of foods, integrity of the digestive tract, and our brain function. When we have a leaky gut, we have a leaky brain. Your irritable mind might be caused by your irritable bowel!

Success Story: GERD Solved with Enzymes and Vitamins

The medical term for heartburn is gastroesophageal reflux disease (GERD). However, GERD is not a disease. For more details, see my article titled, "Acid reflux and Rebellious Stomach: Killing the Messenger for Profit" on my Web site (www.preventionandhealing.com). Also see: "Multiple Patient Success Stories: Positive Responses From Apple Cider Vinegar" on page 186.

This patient's story will help all those who have been told that they need to take medication for their heartburn:

Just wanted to update you... Came to you when regular doctors felt I had GERD and wanted me on Prevacid. You prescribed vitamins, digestive enzymes, and a couple other natural supplements.

Within a few months, I was feeling much better, and now it is rare that I ever have stomach acid problems. I weighed 202 pounds when I first came in. I now weigh 180. The pounds fell off this past summer!

I still occasionally take digestive enzymes, especially if I have had a large meal, and take supplemental vitamins, but not daily. Also, I did add a probiotic this summer. That was the cincher for stopping the GERD and losing weight.

Thanks!

B.H.

Success Story: Pancreatitis and Abdominal Pain Relieved

Pancreatitis is inflammation of the pancreas that can either be acute (sudden) or chronic (long lasting). Chronic pancreatitis usually causes persistent abdominal pain and difficulties with digestion. Because the pancreas plays an important role in digestion, inflammation (or infection) can cause a disturbance in the production of two main substances:

• Digestive juices (enzymes and bicarbonate that neutralize acids)

• Digestive hormones (insulin and glucagon that control blood sugar)

The following section contains my clinical notes about a female patient who suffered from pancreatitis and its side effects for many years:

Chief Complaint: Sara, a 61-year-old female complained of abdominal pain. She had a history of gallstones embedded in her pancreas. She developed adult onset diabetes in 1993. She previously had cholecystectomy (removal of the gallbladder). She previously had an appendectomy and a hysterectomy.

Diagnostics: EDS (electrodermal screening), hair mineral analysis, food allergy tests

Physical Exam: Sara had one amalgam and multiple scars from previous operations. She had abdominal pain upon palpation especially in the upper right quadrant and the epigastric areas.

Results: EDS revealed major disturbances in the gallbladder, stomach, liver, small intestine, spleen, and allergy meridians. It also revealed electro-signals for parasites. Hair mineral analysis revealed aluminum toxicity. Food allergy tests revealed allergies to turkey, pork, shrimp, lobster, and mushroom.

Treatments: I recommended a prescription parasite remedy along with natural parasite-cleansing remedies. Neural therapy (injections of local anesthetics into the scars) was used to reduce the pain from scar tissue from her operations. A rotation diet, based on food allergy test results, was recommended.

Outcome: Sara's abdominal pain was totally relieved. Previously, due to her pain, Sara had severely restricted her diet. Now she can eat with just a few restrictions in her diet. Sara's pancreatitis was relieved.

Summary: Only three injections of the neural therapy were required. Neural therapy is an effective way of reestablishing energy flows along the meridians that have been disturbed by scar tissue. (See: an explanation of neural therapy on the Web page titled "About the Practice".)

Notes

17

Lazarus Effects
(Nervous System
–Related Problems)

I feel positive energy rising within me—
something that had been so depleted by the
effects of mercury poisoning.
S.J.B. (Patient)

S everal times in my book, I have mentioned how I am often
confronted with patients who arrive in my office with a long
list of complaints and a long list of doctors who were unable to
diagnose their problems (including the Mayo clinic). I know that they
have overlooked these five common underlying problems:

- Heavy-metal toxicity

- Food allergies

- Dental problems (often hidden)

- Parasites

- Poor diet and nutrition

I have grouped the patients with mystery illnesses in this chapter with
nervous system related problems. Many of yesterday's "mystery illnesses" have been given new names, such as attention deficit disorder (ADD),
brain fog, and fibromyalgia, to name just a few. Readers will immediately
notice that this group is nervous system–related. Depression, anxiety,

and numerous other wide-spread psychiatric problems may also be grouped in this category.

While mainstream medicine continues to search for the right drug to treat nervous system–related illness, I search for informational clues that may have led to immune system deterioration. If you can correct the underlying problem, it causes a profound shift that enables the body to heal itself. I call this the "Lazarus Effect."

Success Story: Memory Problems Disappear

This case study relays how much mercury poisoning can affect a person's memory. Although this patient also experienced dizziness, headaches, and back pain, memory loss was a threat to her work as a spiritual counselor.

Researchers who have worked with mercury have been providing the world with warnings about mercury's effect on memory since the 1920s. Dr. Alfred Stock, a Professor of Chemistry at the Kaiser Wilhelm Institute in Berlin, became very sick from working with mercury. His April 1926 paper, titled "The Danger of Mercury Vapour," warned anyone involved with mercury during their work. He wrote, "For almost 25 years, I experienced increasing ailments, which sometimes became unbearable to the point that I doubted I would be able to continue my scientific work. However, no doctor succeeded in discovering the reason for this condition. The symptoms were: mental dullness, exhaustion, lack of motivation, and inability to work—particularly intellectually. The most depressing condition was loss of memory. This continually worsened, so that eventually I came close to total memory loss."

Dear Dr. Yu and Staff,

For several weeks I have wanted to write and share the good news of my renewed energy. I am convinced it is related to the gradual removal of mercury from my system, which you and your staff accomplished. Let me share some of the differences I'm experiencing.

Three years ago Christmas, I met you for the first time. I can remember walking into your office feeling very anxious and wondering what I was getting myself into. After my initial surprise when you asked to check my fingers and feet (I was expecting something of a regular physical exam!), I began to realize I was a partner in my own healing. Before this, I often felt like the doctor would heal me. Now I realized you were naming your own hopes and limitations, inviting me to become an active participant in my own healing process. As tests confirmed my mercury level was extremely high (230), I was unfocused, lacked energy, experienced many sinus infections each season, sore throats were common, with upper back pain and pounding headaches adding to my discomfort. I felt I was losing my mind and often lost my balance, walking in odd ways, almost feeling a "disconnect" between my legs and the rest of my body. I was dropping things, forever forgetting where I put things, etc. The simplest tasks seemed impossible.

At this time, you suggested I get an evaluation from Dr. Michael Rehme, DDS, who confirmed your diagnosis that the 13 fillings in my teeth were probably the source of my problem. When I had mentioned to my former dentist that I was concerned about the mercury, he trivialized my fears and assured me there was nothing harmful in mercury fillings. I wonder where I'd be today if I had listened to him? After your evaluation and the subsequent replacement of all 13 fillings, I have noticed a remarkable change in myself. Recently I have given presentations to groups (50 - 60 people) with a minimum of anxiety, being able to focus and sustain thought patterns in questions from participants. I could not do this 3 years ago when I first began this process.

I also feel positive energy rising within me, something that had been so depleted by effects of the mercury poisoning. My attempts to compensate for the inability to focus led to extreme exhaustion. Now I find energy increasing as I research a topic, follow through in creating novel ways to present an idea, and do all the administrative tasks needed. An example of this new energy took place this past Saturday, when I met with 60 school sisters of Notre Dame to discuss the topic: "The Lewis and Clark Expedition as a Metaphor of the Motherhouse Renovation." It was fun, energizing for the sisters, and gave them much food for thought. At the end of the presentation, I felt their positive energy and have been invited to return and explore the topic further.

My primary ministry is that of Spiritual Direction, and my office is at Maria Center, St Louis. Before my treatment for mercury poisoning, I was beginning to feel unable to continue this ministry. It demands careful attention to the feelings underlying the statements an individual might make, and the ability to reflect back what the person has said and where the Spirit might be leading. Due to the exhaustion and pain I previously felt, it was a constant battle to stay attentive to the individual. In a previous instance of consulting a medical doctor, I had been told I would probably be on tranquilizers for the rest of my life. Thank God I sought another opinion.

Now that my mercury count is 26, I find renewed energy to walk into areas of a person's fears in ways that are freeing for the individual and allow God's Spirit to use me in a whole new way. Others are seeing something new in the way I've been "directing" them, and there is new growth possible because I am more in touch with the inner dynamic (gift of the Spirit) known as discernment.

I realize that my recovery has also included a change in diet and nutrition, greater fidelity to exercise (walking and yoga), more rest, focusing less on a filled calendar than times for Shabbat rest, and a steady diet of good reading, good music, and good friends. I am no longer trying to handle difficulties alone, toughing it out as before, but instead am being a vital part of my parish community, my religious community, and my broader Franklin County community. Quality time for prayer and solitude are a "must" for the kind of ministry I offer, and I honor that reality more than ever before. And I continue to see a chiropractor whose philosophy supports your own.

As I consider how I've changed over the past 3 years, I must admit it was a difficult road at times. I would receive chelation therapy from your staff, feeling depleted of any energy at all and then often go to Dr. Rehme's office for dental work. Sometimes I would drive home wondering if I could do it. But both your staff and Dr. Rehme's were so personally supportive and affirming. I remember how you helped me through an especially difficult time by listening without judgment and helping me learn to trust what my body was trying to tell me. I remember how often Ann helped me by her compassionate patience as veins would give out or I would just be weary of the whole process, and how supportive Kate was with each step in my journey. That kindness kept me coming back and seeing the process through to the end.

Finally, this whole process has taught me how threatening your approach must be to the AMA. Only once did I receive a prescription for a drug, amoxicillin, after an especially difficult sinus infection. Yes, the initial cost was expensive, and I wondered if my community could afford it. However, when I look at the benefits, I see the whole process as an investment in better health in the future. I wonder what disease might have developed in me due to the mercury poisoning. MS? cancer, etc.? The whole experience has made me even more a believer in alternative medicine.

To say I am grateful is an understatement. You and Dr. Rehme have given me my life back, and I will never forget your professional expertise and your personal kindness. The "Lazarus" in me says THANK YOU.

S.J.B.

Success Story: Fibromyalgia Disappears

This first case study was written as an e-mail to a friend and copied to me. Besides fibromyalgia, this patient also had chronic fatigue and arthritis pain.

Fibromyalgia has been called a "chronic disorder." In the late 1990s, the National Fibromyalgia Association (NFA) was formed to "improve the quality of life of those with fibromyalgia" and the *British Journal of Rheumatology* published a Norwegian population study of the incidence of fibromyalgia in women 26 to 55 years old and found it to be 583 in 100,000 or 5.8 percent (*Br J Rheumatol.* Dec 1997;36 (12):1318-1323). In June 2006, the *Journal of Clinical Rheumatology* published an American study titled, "The incidence of Fibromyalgia and its associated comorbidities: A population-based retrospective cohort study based on international classification of disease" and found the U.S. occurrence rate to be about 4.2 percent (Peter T. Weir, M.D., et al, June 2006). Would the NFA and the international journals of rheumatology want to know about the factors that lead to immune system deterioration?

Dear M,

First, I Just wanted to THANK YOU, thank you, thank you! for refer-ring me to Dr. Yu. I have seen him twice, and I feel 75% better than I did 3 months ago.

He treated me with every viral, bacterial medicine he had. Said he had never seen so many viral issues with one person. He dewormed, "de-parisited" me, gave me supplements, and I took every one of them with a prayer "let this be the thing that will rid my body of fibromyalgia, chronic fatigue, and the swelling, inflammation, and arthritis pain.... this awful thing that has stolen 4 years of my life."

Since seeing him, I have weaned myself off the steroids, Prednisone, Wellbutrin for my arthritic pain, and the Adderall for energy in the past 4 weeks. Now all I am taking is my thyroid medicine. You don't know how happy that makes me just getting off of those 3 drugs. I have always been an antisynthetic drug person, and it just killed me to have to take those to be able to function every day.

I am also sleeping much better, have an appetite again, which I haven't had for 4 years. Dr. Yu did say he was going to get me fixed up, but not overnight, "and no guarantees." I was willing to and did try almost anything to feel better in the past 4 years. I am just happy feeling the way I feel today compared to 4 weeks ago. It's like a miracle. Really, that's how much better I feel!!!!

What a blessing you were to come to dinner that night, M, and ask how I was feeling. I had been praying for something to help me find out what was wrong with me. I was really starting to lose hope that I was ever going to feel young again and thought I'd be a 40-year-old forever trapped inside an 80-year-old body.

I have always been a very active, physically strong person and enjoyed playing tennis, soccer, and running. I just felt my life had been taken away from me as I was barely able to walk or open a bottle of ketchup. I was very angry and mad that my health had diminished so quickly and that I was expected to keep taking more drugs to numb all the pain that was supposedly in my brain.

M_k has mentioned to me several times that you had called, and that you had asked about my seeing Dr. Yu. I just wanted to take the time to express my deepest gratitude, that this referral to Dr. Yu was the greatest gift anyone could have ever given me.

Today, I got up at 6 AM and D and I walked up that hill in our neighborhood to play tennis for 2 hours, and walked home. I never thought I would be able to do that again!

Thank you, Dr. Yu, for your gifts, talents, knowledge, and study of alternative medicine. I have seen many doctors, taken many medicines, and traveled many miles to the Cleveland Clinic in Ohio, trying to find someone that was able to help me, and to believe me that it was not "all in my head."

I feel like I have my life back again, and I am going to enjoy it for the next 40 years, doing all the things I love to do! Thank you, M and Dr. Yu, and may God bless you both!

I am really looking forward to my next appointment. Now if we could just get me to lose those extra 30 lbs I have gained in the past 4 years (maybe in 3 weeks?). That would be a miracle. I'm working on it.

Dr. Yu, you are more than welcome to put this out there. I am happy to tell everyone why I am feeling so much better. We moved into a new home 4 years ago, and I love to plant flowers and work in my yard. I have not been able to do that since we have moved.

I have been working out in the yard on my landscaping and installed lights in the last 2 weeks. All my neighbors are in awe. They seem to be reacting: "What has gotten into you?" I told them I have energy and feel good again, thanks to Dr. Yu, this new Doctor I have been seeing.

My husband told me last night, "You seem much happier lately." My response is: "Duh!" I feel good! It makes a big difference to wake up feeling good, not tired, and energetic. I feel like I am alive again! So, yes, let everyone know about how you have helped me. I am telling everyone I know about you and what a wonderful Doctor you are!

D.D.

Success Story: Depression and Anger Disappears

The mercuryexposure.org Web site is a volunteer project with the following mission:

> To prevent and reduce mercury exposure in the areas of dentistry, medicine, living environment, and the biosphere, in a humanitarian effort to preserve quality of life.

One of the articles on the site explains that mercury is the root of depression, anger, anxiety, and violence.

The following letter from a female patient describes depression and anger that she realized were caused by the metal in her mouth:

Four years ago, my husband left college with no job or insurance and the three of us moved back to my hometown to rent a small house from my Mom. Within 30 days of having 6 teeth treated with amalgam fillings, I became depressed, angry, and unhappy with a 6-year marriage. At 46, my menstrual cycle was "off," so I thought it must be hormone related. I purchased a book at a very reputable health food store in our community, and that's when the healing process started.

Thinking I needed saliva testing, I called a lab in the book's appendix. They recommended a doctor in St. Louis. Well, he tested my mouth, but not the saliva. The result was a shocking amount of electric current being produced by 12 molars (all with amalgam fillings, i.e., mercury). Reviewing my medical history provided a lot of insight. I had suffered with many illnesses associated with mercury poison: from acne and rheumatoid arthritis to hypoglycemia and low thyroid (just to name a few). And now it was a mental struggle to home-school my son, run a home, stay active in church, maintain my appearance, control my anger, and, in general, just live life. My doctor did a hair analysis and a DMPS. My mercury level excretion was almost 5 times higher than normal. He also gave me lots to read and recommended seeing a biological dentist for mercury removal.

John 8:32, And you shall know the truth, and the truth shall make you free. Healing was going to be all three: spiritually, mentally, and physically. I trusted the Lord to provide the dentist and the finances, since He had already led me to one doctor. My husband and family were skeptical, but I provided them with lots of information. I also talked to a couple in another state who had gone through this. Finally, my dentist discussed the plan for my mouth. I wanted to do it immediately, but that did not happen. In the process of removing the mercury, the metal posts in the two front teeth became infected and a root canal started giving me problems. They had to go, too.

It has been 3 years, and we have just about completed my dental procedures. It took supplements and dental work to rid my body of the mercury. The healing didn't come overnight, but I noticed changes in chunks. About every 3 or 4 months, I would think: "Hey, I feel better!" I haven't been sick, depressed, or yelled at anyone. My energy level is high and, most of all, my husband and son have noticed an improvement. Exercise and a healthy diet have been a part of my life for over 20 years. I've weighed the same since high school, took first place in a bodybuilding contest at 30, and was able to do natural childbirth at 41. But little did I know that the run-of-the-mill dental care was my enemy. We have improved our diet and habits, and now look forward to a longer, healthier life. Thank you, Doctors Yu and Rehme.

C.V.

Success Story: Irritability Gone, Return of Stamina and Energy

Besides anger, depression, and anxiety, irritability and brain fog are also symptoms of mercury toxicity. This patient noticed that he felt less irritable when his amalgams were removed.

The most obvious change for me was the return of stamina and energy. I felt like my old self. However, as I went through the checklist, I also realized that irritability that I had associated with stress has all but disappeared. That realization makes great sense to me because the stress has not decreased.

C.C.

Success Story: ADD and ADHD Disappear

ADD and ADHD are abbreviations for attention-deficit disorder and attention-deficit hyperactivity disorder.

These problems are so widespread, thousands of parents across the country are forming support groups. Many of the groups are online. Yahoo groups lists 584 attention-deficit groups, and many have thousands of members. Most parents are so conditioned to search for drug solutions, many members discuss where to buy psychiatric drugs, such as Adderall and Ritalin.

One of the biggest concerns about ADHD drugs is their side effects. These drugs have potentially serious side effects, such as high blood pressure, irregular heart beat, and dependency. In July 2009, a CBS television news story said that as many as 25 percent of college students are taking ADHD drugs to focus. About one third to two thirds of the children with ADHD diagnosed in childhood continue to have symptoms in adult life. The CBS news story said that adult college students who are prescribed ADHD drugs were introducing them to their friends.

The following section contains my clinical notes about a boy who was diagnosed with ADHD and given Ritalin when he was in second grade.

Chief Complaint: Charles, a 12-year-old male, was diagnosed with ADHD in second grade and has been on Ritalin since then. Symptoms include irritability, short fuse, impulsivity, obsessiveness, and constant sugar cravings.

Diagnostics: EDS (electrodermal screening), hair mineral analysis, food allergy test

Physical Exam: Normal

Results: Hair mineral analysis revealed an inverted sodium/potassium ratio indicating adrenal exhaustion. Food allergy testing revealed multiple food allergies to all dairy products, egg, wheat, gluten, and rye.

Treatments: Avoidance of food to which Charles is allergic. Avoid sugar and honey. I suggested a rotation diet based on the food allergy testing. The treatment also included nutritional supplementation based on the results of the hair mineral analysis. Homeopathic remedies were used to balance Charles' metabolism.

Commentary: Charles usually started his day with cereal with honey or sugar along with bacon and eggs. His typical lunch would be a sandwich with cookies. Dinner was typically meat with pasta and bread. Food allergies have commonly been associated with headaches, joint pains, skin rashes, sinus problems, indigestion, depression, achy muscles, fatigue, fluid retention, overweight, and central nervous system disturbances.

A rotation diet consists of totally avoiding allergy-related foods for 6 to 8 weeks. Then gradually the allergy-related foods are reintroduced one at a time on the basis of eating the foods only once every 4 to 5 days.

Outcome: Charles' behavior significantly improved so that he didn't require any Ritalin.

Summary: ADD/ADHD often responds to avoidance of sugars and the elimination diet based on food allergy test results. If heavy-metal toxicity is involved, the symptoms of ADD/ADHD are more severe, and it will take much longer to reverse the symptoms.

ADD/ADHD has evolved as the new buzzword in today's fast-paced society. Any child with signs of hyperactivity and inattention is in danger of being given the label ADD/ADHD. Such children are at risk for a "blanket prescription" of drugs and psychostimulants, regardless of the underlying causes. There are far too many ADHD look-alike diagnoses that I have described in an in-depth article on my Web site (http:// www.preventionandhealing.com).

Success Story: Anxiety and Depression Disappear

The following section contains my clinical notes about a woman whose story reads like a nightmare suspense saga written for television. At 33, she found herself locked in a psychiatric unit after a dentist put an amalgam filling in her mouth. Although the tension of being locked in a psychiatric unit might be content for television, very few script writers would know, understand, or even be allowed to tell the truth about the cause of many psychiatric problems.

Chief Complaint: Mary, a 33-year-old female, complained of acute episodes of anxiety, depression, and panic attacks. She "escaped" from a locked-in psychiatric unit with her mother, stating that the psychiatric medications were making her feel worse. When I asked about her history, she indicated her problems started one week after she had one large amalgam placed by her dentist. One week later, she was in a psychiatric unit.

Diagnostics: Acupuncture Meridian Assessment, hair mineral analysis, DMPS challenge test for heavy-metal toxicity

Physical Exam: Normal exam except multiple silver fillings (amalgams)

Results: Tests for mercury indicated extremely high mercury toxicity

Treatments: Chelation therapy, detoxification, nutritional therapy

Commentary: Mercury is received from many sources, including silver fillings, air pollution, seafood, cosmetics, and vaccinations. Silver fillings are commonly composed of approximately 50% mercury, 20% silver, 20% copper, and 10% tin. The percentages vary, depending on the specific amalgam.

Treatment: Mary had the one amalgam that started her problems replaced with nonmetal composite material.

Outcome: Within several days after removing this amalgam, she felt greatly improved. Her anxiety, depression, and panic attacks resolved. She was able to return to work, get married on schedule, which was to occur 2 months after the problems began.

Summary: Mary saw me for a total of two visits. She chose only to replace the one amalgam that triggered her problems. She should have continued a total treatment program including removal of all amalgams, cleansing and detoxification of heavy metals, and nutritional support to avoid future problems of the same or different nature.

Often, patients choose only to eliminate the immediate ailment without understanding why they became ill in the first place. There are often multiple causes that lead to illness that must be fully resolved in order to avoid other illness in the future. It is the elimination of causes that weaken the psycho-neuro-endocrine and immune system that allow the body's healing to occur and improves one's health. One of the most common causes of psychiatric problems, of which most medical doctors are unaware, is heavy-metal toxicity.

Success Story: Chronic Fatigue, Fibromyalgia, and MS-Like Symptoms

The Professional Guide to Diseases, now in its 8th edition, contains this information about multiple sclerosis (MS):

> The exact cause of MS is unknown, but current theories suggest a slow-acting or latent viral infection and an auto-immune response. Other theories suggest that environmental and genetic factors may also be linked to MS. Emotional stress, overwork, fatigue, pregnancy, and acute respiratory tract infections have been known to precede the onset of this illness.

For political reasons, mercury poisoning is a subject that never appears in the American media including books. The few books that exist have been self-published by dentists who have had the courage to confront the American Dental Association, which denies that mercury amalgams are toxic. Dr. Hal Huggins is an example, and his book, *It's All in Your Head: The Link Between Mercury Amalgams and Illness* is sold in health food stores. He is also coauthor of *Uninformed Consent: The Hidden Dangers in Dental Care*. In 1996,

Huggins lost his license for refusing to place, or recommend placing, silver amalgams and refusing to recommend or place root canals. He has multiple sclerosis (MS) and has consistently witnessed improvement in MS patients undergoing amalgam removal.

Gerald Hendess, a German researcher who wrote a paper called, "Multiple sclerosis, some considerations concerning MS," says that mercury as the cause of MS is ignored completely. In his paper, he explains that MS was first described by Cruveilhier in 1835 and only seems to have existed for less than the past 200 years. He also explains that it was around this time that people in Europe first had their teeth filled with amalgam, initially in England and then in France. Hendess writes:

> *This rather exact chronological correspondence with the beginning of the MS disease could be a pure coincidence. However there are further indications that lead to amalgam. Observations have been made that MS occurs more often in industrialized countries than in third-world countries. Until now there is no commonly accepted explanation. Amalgam could fill this explanation gap quite easily.*

The following section contains my clinical notes about a woman who developed multiple sclerosis-like symptoms.

Chief Complaint: Peggy, a 50-year-old female registered nurse, came to see me in March 2000 complaining of chronic fatigue, fibromyalgia, and multiple sclerosis-like symptoms. Peggy complained of weakness of her left foot, dragging this foot with sensations of electrical vibrations in her leg. Her body movements were jerky, and she suffered sharp pains all over. Her neurologist suspected Peggy might have multiple sclerosis (MS); a spinal tap and MRI were performed. The spinal tap and MRI were negative; they did not show any sign of

---

British Press Is More Open to the Truth About Mercury Toxicity Than the American Press

The British press is often more conscientious about truthful reporting than the American press. In November 2004, the BBC aired a story titled, "Woman Blames Mercury for Depression" about a woman who suffered from depression for four decades, spending much of the time in a British mental institution. The woman's family and friends persuaded the hospital to allow her to visit a dentist to have her mercury amalgams removed in January 2004, and she was discharged from the hospital ten months later.

MS. The neurologist recommended that Peggy wait for another spinal tap and MRI the following year. Peggy knew something was obviously wrong with her, so she decided to seek a second opinion, rather than just stand idly by waiting for another year to pass.

Diagnostics: Acupuncture Meridian Assessment, galvanic current evaluation, hair mineral analysis, DMPS chelation challenge test for heavy-metal toxicity

Physical Exam: Unremarkable exam, except 9 amalgams plus multiple crowns and varicose veins. Neurological exam was unremarkable.

Results: EDS showed disturbances to Peggy's dental meridians. It also showed disturbances to her kidney and bladder meridians. She was taking antibiotics at the time for a urinary tract infection. The nerve system showed a disturbance only to the left side of her body, indicating an asymmetry in her meridian system consistent with her clinical symptoms. Her left adrenal meridian also showed a weakness consistent with chronic fatigue symptoms.

Galvanic current was very high. This has been known to disturb autonomic nervous system function. Hair mineral analysis revealed extremely high aluminum toxicity. DMPS chelation challenge test revealed extremely high mercury toxicity and also a high tin toxicity.

Treatments: I recommended that Peggy have her amalgams replaced. An herbal body cleansing program was started along with nutritional supplementation, based on the results of the hair mineral analysis.

Commentary: The galvanic current is measured in the mouth in very small amounts using units of millivolts and microamperes. It measures the "mouth battery" that is created by electrical currents between various metals in and on the teeth, and the saliva that conducts the current. It causes irritations in the nervous system and releases the heavy metal at a fast rate from the amalgam into the tissues in the oral cavity and the rest of the body.

Outcome: One year later, Peggy's follow-up exam showed that she had part of her amalgams replaced. She stated that she was feeling much better. Her neurological symptoms had all essentially disappeared, except when she is very tired. She lost 40 pounds based on my dietary recommendations. Peggy's husband stated, "I got my wife back." Peggy promised to complete her amalgam replacement.

Part 5

My Crock Pot Ideas

Notes

18

Crock Pot Ideas?

Quality in everyday life can be achieved by slowing down, respecting the traditions of the table and celebrating the diversity of the Earth's bounty.
- Slow Food USA

When I first started using the expression "crock pot idea," I used it as a warning to my readers—that my ideas were not totally aligned with the medical establishment. At first, the ideas stirred up reactions very similar to the crock pot's reception in the 1970s, 80s, and 90s. For some, a crock pot made from stone represented a time-saving appliance, but most people could not relate to gentle, slow cooking. All that has changed now that "slow food" is better understood. There are "gourmet" slow cooker cook books, and there's even a "slow food" movement in Europe and the United States. Similarly, ideas that were once thought to be extreme in medicine are now widely accepted.

In this chapter, you'll find a collection of my "crock pot ideas" that were published in *The Healthy Planet* magazine.

80% Solution for 20% of the Problem: What a Crock Pot Idea!

My crock pot idea expression began with this article that explains my approach to treatment.

❧ ❧ ❧

People often come to see me with a fixed idea for a specific treatment as if they have already made their own diagnosis. They are looking for a doctor who will listen to them. They want a doctor who will follow their lead and solve what they think are their unique medical problems because they feel that they have already been misdiagnosed and mistreated by numerous medical doctors.

In a typical scenario, a middle-aged, well-educated female patient will come to see me with a complaint of chronic fatigue and mood disorder (that she has had for many years). This same patient typically has normal hormone and blood tests but has been told that she is depressed and may need antianxiety/antidepressive medication.

Thanks to the Internet, this same patient has done research on holistic/alternative medical therapies and knows that a blood test may not match clinical symptoms. She is convinced that she is suffering from subclinical hypothyroidism, adrenal fatigue, and hormonal imbalance with a chronic yeast infection and hidden allergies.

This type of patient also provides me with a "treatment plan" that starts with antifungal medication and a yeast-free diet, followed by low-dose natural thyroid medication, adrenal glandular support, and estrogen/progesterone replacement therapy. She also knows that she needs a tissue mineral analysis, a food allergy test, a saliva hormone profile, and possibly a dental evaluation for amalgams. What she wants is a physician who understands all these approaches to health problems—a physician who will coordinate their care.

I have had some great success with some of the most challenging medical conditions. However, every case is unique. I'm trained not to listen to a "self-diagnosis and treatment plan," but to go back to a basic, individualized evaluation.

My initial evaluation encompasses a detailed medical history, a physical exam, an Acupuncture Meridian Assessment, and basic lab tests including a hair mineral analysis, a food allergy test, and a hormone evaluation if indicated.

On the first visit, the basic evaluation gives me the foundation to explore more specific problems. My treatment plan may contradict what the patient has in his/her "treatment plan." Once in a while, I get a message that a patient is not coming back for a follow-up visit because "the doctor is not listening to their complaints." Apparently, I am too ignorant to understand such a patient's self-diagnosis and treatment plan.

Why do we get sick? What does it take to get well? The answers are complex issues that cannot be fully addressed in one visit. I always encourage people to search my Web site for specific topics and to read the success stories. I also encourage patients to attend my free monthly lecture that provides a broader view of my holistic approach to prevention and healing.

The most important part of my treatment plan starts with patient education about what it means to view life holistically and to understand the biology of man. I strongly believe that the body has an innate healing capacity. It will always attempt to heal itself.

I also encourage patients and readers to start thinking of the human body as a fine musical instrument. A violin is a good example because when it is out of tune, it starts making a funny noise. The funny noise is the equivalent of symptoms, such as aches and pains, fatigue, anxiety, or depression.

My job as a physician is to try to balance meridians that have been out of tune for some time. After tuning the violin (in this case, the body), it is up to you to determine how well you want to play. How we think, eat, exercise, and play is up to an individual. We all have a unique style of playing music called "life." We play solo, in a duet (a husband and wife), in a quartet (a family), and in a symphony of life.

I also like to use a cooking metaphor with my patients. By the time people come to see me, they may have at least 10 major underlying issues and problems. Out of 10, I might be able to modify only 5 major problems. Those that are modifiable are environmental toxins, such as mercury or lead toxicity, food allergies, parasites, hidden infections, nutritional deficiencies, and a need for general detoxification. The other 5 problems are beyond my ability to correct, such as genetic makeup, early childhood physical and emotional traumas, scars and vaccinations, dental problems, or religious and family dynamics. Metaphorically, a patient's major problems are like cooking ingredients. You have a cooking pot, but you only get to choose 5 of the 10 ingredients.

Realistically, I might be able to fix only 80 percent of the 5 modifiable problems. That translates into an 80 percent solution for 20 percent of the original problems. I hope my math is not too confusing.

One of the most important steps is prioritizing the problems. We must look for a specific, modifiable, common denominator that influences an imminent problem. Your body will start responding to the rest of the problems as the body heals itself.

Comparing the human body to a violin and then a cooking pot seems like a rather wacky idea. The water in the pot is like emotion that holds the essence of life. How we stir the pot gives us the final unique flavor of an individual human. I better stop! There are a lot of crock pot ideas in medicine. Searching for more metaphors begins to sound more like another crock pot idea!

Lyme Disease Under the Limelight: Is It Really a Hidden Dental Problem?

In this article, I explain some of the stumbling blocks related to Lyme disease tests and the dangers of overdiagnosing Lyme disease.

ૐ ૐ ૐ

Lyme disease and Lyme arthritis were first recognized in 1975 in the region of Lyme, Connecticut. The discovery of Lyme resulted from an unusual cluster of children experiencing arthritic pain after developing skin lesions with a bull's-eye red rash called erythema chronicum migrans. Lyme disease is a tick-borne inflammatory disorder caused by a relatively newly recognized spirochete, *Borrelia burgdorferi*, isolated by Dr. Willy Burgdorfer.

The classical symptom of the skin lesions with a bull's-eye red rash is followed weeks to months later by neurologic, cardiac, or joint pains. The primary carriers of Lyme disease are tiny nymphs called Ixodid ticks. Now we know that the bull's eye is not a necessary symptom and that Lyme disease may be spread in several ways and not just through ticks. The rising incidence of Lyme disease in recent years in the United States may be explained by an exploding deer population and outward expansion of suburban homes into wooded rural areas. Lyme disease is also widely present in Europe, Asia, and other continents.

The latest medical hypothesis indicates that Lyme disease is linked to over 300 diseases, including fibromyalgia, chronic fatigue syndrome, Parkinson's disease, multiple sclerosis (MS), amyotrophic lateral sclerosis (ALS), brain fog, dilated cardiomyopathy, anxiety, and a wide spectrum of physical and psychiatric dysfunctions. The good news is that all stages of Lyme disease may respond to *appropriate* antibiotic treatment.

Is Lyme disease a new hidden epidemic or pandemic disease that has not been recognized? Is Lyme ignored by the medical and scientific community? If Lyme disease is so common, why isn't this debilitating disease readily recognized? The crux of the problem is the reliability of the laboratory test for Lyme disease.

There are three main diagnostic tests currently available for Lyme disease: the Lyme enzyme–linked immunosorbent assay (ELISA) screening test, the Western blot, and the Lyme polymerase chain reaction (PCR) test. Additional lab tests include Lyme dot assay from a urine sample, the Lyme C6 peptide ELISA, and the CD57 lymphocyte subset test. Unfortunately, there is massive confusion among Lyme disease experts when it comes to interpreting laboratory results. The controversy surrounding laboratory test results creates problems for doctors who try to diagnose and treat Lyme disease.

In February 2005, I attended a Lyme disease conference and felt compelled to notify the public that Lyme disease may be a new buzzword and fad to explain mysterious and chronic debilitating illnesses. The latest *rapid* test for diagnosing Lyme disease is called the Bowen/Whitaker quantitative rapid identification of *Borrellia burgdorferi* (Q-RIBb), developed by Jo Anne Whitaker, M.D. This test is "rapid" due to the fact that a report of the laboratory findings is available 24 hours after a blood specimen is received in the laboratory. The test became an overnight sensation in the alternative medical community. But is it accurate?

In my work with patients who have hidden dental infections, I have seen correlations between bacteria infections in the mouth and the diseases that are now labeled Lyme-like (amyotrophic lateral sclerosis, Parkinson's disease, multiple sclerosis, chronic fatigue, heart failure, and others I have mentioned earlier in this article).

Polymerase Chain Reaction (PCR) Test Has an Interesting History

Although a polymerase chain reaction (PCR) test is not practical for diagnosing Lyme disease, it has become a useful tool in law enforcement and paternity testing. Archaeologists also use it to determine evolutionary relationships among organisms.

The polymerase chain reaction is a molecular biology technique for duplicating a DNA sequence into millions of copies. The "dawn of the age of PCR" occurred when a chemist named Kary Mullis was driving in his car with his girlfriend. They were both employed as chemists at Cetus Corporation and, during their drive, Kary came up with an idea that would duplicate DNA an infinite number of times. Mullis spent more than a year trying to perfect the technique and succeeded on December 16, 1983. Cetus gave him a $10,000 bonus for his invention.

Spirochete infections in the mouth are caused by a different species than the species that cause Lyme disease. Apparently, the news that these vastly different spirochete species share common antigen proteins has not reached the alternative medical community. A study that describes this shortcoming in Lyme testing was published in the *Journal of Clinical Microbiology* (See: "Spirochete Family Shares Proteins That Can Trigger False-Positive Test Results for Lyme Disease"). The researchers' findings confirm my suspicion that common proteins are confusing the interpretation of Whitaker's Q-RIBb test for Lyme.

Dr. Whitaker has had Lyme disease since childhood and her dissatisfaction with Lyme tests led her to develop a test that looks for the Bb organism. Her test uses a fluorescent staining technique to identify the antigen of the cystic or L-form (cell-wall–deficient form) of the bacteria in the blood bacteria, and not the body's antibodies. Note: For a detailed explanation of the words antigen and antibody, see: "Sorting Out the Meaning of the Words Antibody and Antigen."

Dr. Lida Mattman, a prominent microbiologist who was nominated for a Nobel Prize for her work on stealth pathogens in 1997, has supported Whitaker's test results because she has cultured Lyme bacteria from its cell-wall–deficient form (cystic or L-form) to spirochetes in a laboratory. Although Mattman's work has confirmed the presence of the *Borrelia burgdorferi* from blood samples that have been screened using the Whitaker Q-RIBb test for Lyme, the cultures that Dr. Mattman developed *were only for Mattman studies.*

In one Mattman study, Lyme Q-RIBb disease tests showed all fibromyalgia patients tested were positive for Lyme disease. Whitaker and Mattman even go so far as to say that all samples from the general population tested with the Lyme Q-RIBb are positive for Lyme.

Whitaker and Mattman have been acknowledged for their test's ability to identify a cystic form of *Borrelia Burgdorferi*, which is the hardest to kill. Cystic forms are covered by a thickened external membrane that helps the *Borrelia burgdorferi* survive antibiotic treatments and adverse environmental conditions inside or outside the body.

The Whitaker data creates a major dilemma and conflict when it comes to understanding Lyme diagnostic tests. How could everyone test positive for Lyme disease? *All* spirochetes, including *Borrelia burgdorferi*, have been known to undergo a pleomorphic cycle of cystic and granular variant forms depending on the environment. Pleomorphism is a concept that I first described in Chapter Two in a section titled "The Health of the Body's Internal Environment." It refers to the occurrence of 2 or more structural forms during an organism's life cycle. With this in mind, it is important to remember that the Q-RIBb test for Lyme may be overidentifying cysts because all spirochete species form cysts.

Some of my chronically ill patients have gone to Lyme disease specialists and have been diagnosed with the Q-RIBb test. They were

---

Sorting Out the Meaning of the Words Antibody and Antigen

Unless you use the words antibody and antigen regularly, the subject of a possible false-positive Lyme test may still be confusing.

An antigen is a substance that triggers the immune system to produce an antibody. Antigens are usually proteins or polysaccharides derived from bacteria, viruses, protozoans, microorganisms, or larger parasites, such as worms. Antigens may be from the outer surfaces of a cell (capsular antigens), from the cell interior (the somatic or O antigens), or from the flagella (the flagellar or H antigens). In the *Journal of Clinical Microbiology* study, the researchers discovered flagellar proteins that were common to different spirochete species, including the *Borrelia burgdorferi*. Note: A flagella is a spirochete's long, threadlike extension, which functions as an organ of locomotion. All spirochetes have this appendage.

also given intravenous antibiotics for extensive periods of time. I am quite alarmed by such aggressive antibiotic therapy. Is Lyme disease frequently misdiagnosed or overdiagnosed? Are we treating for the wrong reasons and are some people getting well accidentally? These are very important questions to be addressed.

I believe there are 2 distinct diseases: Lyme disease caused by *Borrelia burgdorferi* and a Lyme disease–like syndrome (Lyme complex) caused by many other underlying problems. Lyme disease caused by *Borrelia burgdorferi* belongs to the spirochete family. Syphilis is a well-known disease caused by a spirochete called *Treponema pallidum.* The spirochete is a very common oral microorganism that is associated with root canals, dental abscesses, and cavitations. Spirochetes have also been known to cause:

- Carditis (inflammation of the heart)
- Neuropathy (deranged function of the peripheral nerves)
- Fibromyalgia (chronic widespread body pain and a painful response to pressure)
- Severe fatigue

Note: For details about Dr. Weston Price's discovery of a connection between spirochetes and degenerative disease, see: "Spirochete Family Shares Proteins That Can Trigger False-Positive Test Results for Lyme Disease."

Heavy metals, environmental toxins, parasites, and unrecognized dental infections can create conditions for a relatively benign spirochete bacteria to transform into an aggressive pathogen that can cause symptoms mimicking Lyme disease. Syphilis has been known as a "great imitator" because its symptoms can mimic so many other clinical manifestations. Now, Lyme disease seems to be taking over the title of great imitator. Chronically ill patients who have been diagnosed with Lyme disease can have over 300 different symptoms!

It is imperative to understand that there is a Lyme disease and a Lyme disease–like syndrome. Otherwise, our medical and scientific community will be marching into an intellectually dead-end solution for Lyme and Lyme-like illness. Overdiagnosis of Lyme disease will only lead to a "one-disease-fits-all," dead-end antibiotic treatment plan. Treatment should always be individualized and not be dependent on lab test results alone. One should always look for other underlying medical conditions and cofactors, such as hidden

Even the Mainstream Media Questions the Long-Term Antibiotic Therapy Given to Lyme Patients

The most dangerous aspect of a false-positive test result for Lyme disease is the long-term antibiotic therapy that always follows.

Although the mainstream media rarely questions drug therapy, in July 2008, *ABC News* interviewed the Chief of Infectious Diseases at New York Medical College who said, "long-term antibiotic therapy has not proven effective and may be dangerous."

Although the *ABC News* report weighed heavily in favor of antibiotic therapy saying it is "worth the risk," the story refers to "the long-term medication debate" and says organizations such as the Infectious Diseases Society have agreed to review its governing guidelines for Lyme disease.

dental infections, heavy metals, parasites, nutritional deficiency, and environmental toxins.

Lyme disease and spirochete infection are the latest "culprits" in the limelight. It is imperative that medical practitioners review the whole person while searching for multiple causative factors of illness. We should not be too quick to simply look for the "one" culprit that may be found in the latest attention-grabbing headline.

Lyme Disease Diagnosis in Dogs Is Challenging— Just As It Is in Humans

Canine Lyme disease (CLD) was first identified in Connecticut in 1984, and the number of reported cases has substantially increased since that time. Diagnosis in dogs is as difficult as it is in humans, and the situation is complicated by the fact that veterinarians are administering Lyme disease vaccinations that Tulane University researchers say elicit strong antibody responses, making it difficult to determine a dog's infection status (*Clinical and Diagnostic Laboratory Immunology*, May 2004).

A problem with cross-reactivity of antibodies also exists in dogs as it does in humans. This means that tests for a *Borrelia* organism in a dog may yield a false-positive result because a dog's body may produce the same antibodies in response to *Borrelia* as with other bacterial agents that cause inflammatory disease.

Spirochete Family Shares Proteins That Can Trigger False-Positive Test Results for Lyme Disease

In a study published in the June 1990 issue of the *Journal of Clinical Microbiology* ("Cross reactivity of nonspecific treponemal antibody in serologic tests for Lyme disease"), researchers from Connecticut, California, and Missouri explain that tests for Lyme disease can produce false-positive results because the species of spirochetes that cause Lyme, syphilis, and periodontal disease all share similar proteins that confuse the interpretation of the test results.

In order to understand the potential for a false-positive test result, it is necessary to look at the spirochete family of bacteria and understand their relationship to specific diseases. The following chart lists spirochetes with common antigen proteins that can lead to a false-positive test:

Spirochete	Disease	Notes
Borrelia burgdorferi	Lyme	
Treponema pallidum	Syphilis	
Treponema denticola	Periodontitis	In *Root Canal Cover Up*, Dr. George Meinig says that spirochetes and fusiform bacilli are generally present in most mouths.
Treponema vincentii	Periodontitis	
Treponema socronskii	Periodontitis	
Treponema pectinovorum	Periodontitis	

Disease Transmission

Syphilis is a sexually transmitted disease that can also be acquired congenitally, meaning it can be present at birth. When a disease is present at birth, it can be hereditary or acquired through fetal development. If untreated, syphilis can lead to the degeneration of the heart, bones, and nerve tissue.

Periodontitis is gum disease caused by bacteria that collect in the spaces between the gum and lower part of a tooth's crown. If left unchecked, gum disease can spread to the bones of the jaw.

It is important to realize that the connection between mouth bacteria and degenerative disease has been mostly ignored. Gum disease is the only spirochete-causing oral disease that is acknowledged by modern dental specialists. A significant body of research work by early 20th century dental research specialist, Dr. Weston Price, and his coworking scientists in the fields of bacteriology, pathology, rheumatology, immunology, chemistry, cardiology, and surgery *has been covered up*. At the end of his career, Dr. George Meinig, one of the founding members of the American Association of Endodontists (root canal specialists), summarized 25 years of Price's root canal research in his book, *Root Canal Cover-Up*.

Meinig's book explains that Price was prompted to study the connection between oral infection and degenerative disease when he noticed an extremely large variety of degenerative diseases in patients with root-canal–treated teeth and cavitation infections. Through meticulous research, Price proved that this connection exists. Meinig's detailed 220-page book helps readers understand Price's two volumes that fill more than 1,100 pages.

More than three quarters of a century later, the dentists who are performing approximately 24 million root canal procedures and 20 million extractions each year do not want to hear about the wide range of degenerative illnesses caused by bacteria in root canals or cavitations. Note: Tooth extractions may leave an infected pocket known as a cavitation. In his book, Meinig says, "It will astound most dentists and physicians to learn we have not conquered the infectious organisms in teeth. We believe we control by root canal therapy."

Meinig writes about spirochete bacteria and says, "The influence of spirochete infections upon the health of people can be both severe and rapid." He says spirochetes and fusiform baccilli are "generally present in most mouths, but *become pathogenic when a person becomes debilitated, nutritionally compromised, or badly neglects the care of his or her mouth.*"

Lyme Tests That Measure Antibodies and Antigens
Whether a Lyme test measures antigens or antibodies, if the antigens are common to several different species of spirochetes, then the test results need to be questioned.

Most laboratory tests for Lyme disease look for the presence of an antibody that the body produces in response to the *Borrelia burgdorferi* spirochete. Dr. Jo Anne Whitaker's Q-RIBb test is described as a test that looks for the presence of antigens specific to the *Borrelia burgdorferi* spirochete. However, her test is entirely dependent on antibodies that she fluoresces to visually detect the presence of the *Borrelia burgdorferi* in progressively more dilute blood samples. If she continues to see the fluorescent antibody in very dilute samples, her test confirms the presence of the *Borrelia burgdorferi*. Whitaker calls her test:

> *A titration serial dilution method for quantitating the amount of Bb antigen in the blood.*

The word "quantitate" means to measure or estimate, and the word estimate means approximate.

If several spirochete species share the same protein antigens, then Whitaker may be counting proteins that belong to several different spirochetes, or possibly even other bacteria.

Heavy Cost of Long-Term Antibiotic Therapy
Long-term antibiotic therapy to kill one or more spirochetes is equivalent to dumping toxic chemicals on soil to kill one invading organism. Although the chemical may kill the offending organism, it kills every organism, including the beneficial microbes that help feed nutrients to plants. In the long-term, antibiotics and soil chemicals are the worst possible option for the problem of disease. I consider them to be shortcuts that have devastating results. Throughout my book, I have described multiple underlying problems that are are so widespread in the patient population I have met in my 25 years of practice. Given the fact that I treat patients from all over the country, it makes sense that these underlying problems need to be investigated first—by every physician.

Lupus: Autoimmune Disease and Hidden Pathogens

There are more than 80 diseases caused by autoimmunity—a condition that exists when the body attacks its own cells. Conventional medicine's treatment is medication that decreases the immune response (called immunosuppression).

In this article, I explain how a lupus patient made remarkable progress when 3 major underlying problems were addressed: hidden dental infections, heavy-metal toxicity, and parasite infection.

≥≈ ≥≈ ≥≈

Lupus is a classic case of an autoimmune disease that is described as having *no known cause.* In other words, modern medicine does not have an effective treatment to correct the underlying problems. Because the cause(s) of the disease is unknown, the disease is elusive—baffling both doctors and medical scientists.

An autoimmune disease is one in which one's own antibodies attack one's own cells. As an autoimmune disease, lupus can manifest as inflammation in any organ system, such as the intestinal tract, heart, lung, joints, kidney, or skin. Physicians resort to treating symptoms such as chronic pain and other related clinical manifestations, which result from inflammation. By treating symptoms, and not the underlying problems of the body, the disease itself is not addressed.

Treatment for lupus includes nonsteroidal antiinflammatory drugs (NSAIDs), such as aspirin or ibuprofen, steroids, hydroxychloroquine, and cyclophosphamide. These medications are highly toxic to one's body and create side effects that are, in the long run, more harmful than the original problem.

One of the intriguing aspects of lupus is that some cases respond well to long-term use of antibiotic or antiparasite medications or extraction of an infected root canal.

What is the connection between a hidden infection and autoimmune disease? When you connect the missing links of overlooked scientific studies, one finds indications that hidden infections have been associated not only with lupus, but with most autoimmune diseases such as rheumatoid arthritis, as well as thrombosis, heart attack, and cancer.

Hidden infections seem to be a major culprit causing inflammation and the elevation of the following markers that are hallmarks of autoimmune disease:

- **Erythrocyte sedimentation rate (ESR)**—Erythrocytes are red blood cells, and inflammation causes the protein in red blood cells to clump. Clumping creates dense cells that sink to the bottom of a test tube faster than normal cells. An ESR test, also called sed rate or sedimentation rate, cannot diagnose the condition causing inflammation, but the rate at which the blood cells sink is an indicator of the amount of inflammation in the body.

- **C-reactive protein (CRP)**—a protein found in the blood, which when elevated, reflects inflammation.

- **Antinuclear antibody titre (ANA)**—This test is a measure of the antibodies present in the blood. A titre is the amount that a blood sample can be diluted before the antibodies can no longer be detected. Titre is expressed as a ratio such as 1:40 or 1:80 where a larger second number means that there are more antibodies in the blood. A normal titre is 1:40 or less.

The most prominent scientists who have identified the link between hidden infection and inflammation are Dr. Weston Price in dentistry,

Lida Mattman, Ph.D., in microbiology, and Dr. Gunther Enderlein, Ph.D., in zoology.

Infectious pathogens are often hidden and undetected by standard blood or stool cultures. Depending on environmental stresses, such as root canals, or chronic parasite infestations in the GI tract, pathogens can adapt, change form, and mutate from an overuse of antibiotic medications. A mutated form of a pathogen is often called a cell-wall–deficient form or L form. This mutant becomes a stealth pathogen that is capable of evading our immune surveillance system.

An L-form stealth pathogen is often resistant to antibiotics as well as heat and cold. It can release extreme levels of toxins and be dormant for many years in the body, soil, or refrigerator. An L-form stealth pathogen has different morphology in different stages, depending on the environmental conditions (this is called pleomorphism). Such an organism can create the conditions for chronic medical problems, depending on one's individual genetic susceptibility.

Once an L-form stealth pathogen settles into the body, it can hide in deep cellular levels. Eradicating this type of pathogen can be a major challenge. At this stage, the use of stronger, newer antibiotics creates a bigger monster that must be dealt with later. Stronger antibiotics will only drive a stealth pathogen to become more powerful and more toxic. This will only make the original health problem worse and create symptoms that are more severe.

One of the most effective ways to deal with a stealth pathogen is to reactivate one's immune system through detoxification, nutritional support, and heavy-metal removal, while simultaneously eradicating the pathogen from its hiding places in the GI tract and mouth (in the teeth, gums, and the jaw). The following patient success story illustrates the effectiveness of these strategies. The patient's story is recorded in this excerpt from my clinical notes:

Jane, a 46-year-old female with a history of lupus, arrived in my office in October 2003. Her lupus had been diagnosed in October 1994.

Chief Complaints: Symptoms of recurrent pericarditis (inflammation of the pericardium or the sac surrounding the heart), arthralgia (joint pain), anemia, alopecia (hair loss), pleurisy (inflammation of the lining of the lungs that causes pain), tachycardia (abnormal heart rhythm), fatigue, left shoulder pain, and an elevated ANA.

Physical Exam: Normal

Lab: Electrocardiogram (EKG), normal. Chest x-ray, normal. ANA titre, high with antinuclear antibodies at 1:320. ESR, high at 55. C-reactive protein, very high at 7.13 (a normal value is less than one) and rheumatoid factor, normal at 4. Echocardiogram, normal.

Heavy Metals: Very high level of mercury and slightly elevated level of arsenic and tin

Results: Acupuncture Meridian Assessment (AMA) revealed that the primary problem areas were an intestinal and dental infection.

Treatment: Patient was started on antiparasite medications and antibiotics for her dental infection, even though her dental infection did not bother her. She was also strongly advised to see a biological dentist and given an intensive nutritional program. In April 2004, her dental work was completed by an oral surgeon. Soon after her oral surgery, the patient's aches, chest pain, and pleurisy were resolved. Four months later, her ESR and CRP were back to normal and her ANA titre was down to 1:160.

Commentary: Jane had classic lupus with common physical symptoms and lab test results. Her 3 major underlying problems were hidden dental infections, heavy-metal toxicity, and parasite infection.

Outcome: Jane's chest and joint pain were markedly improved after her intense nutritional program, parasite cleansing, and the completion of her oral surgery for cavitations (infections) in the area of old wisdom teeth sockets. She is going through chelation therapy for heavy-metal toxicity, and I expect she will continue to improve.

In November 2007, Jane's ANA titre was negative, meaning that antibodies were not detectable in her blood. According to RDL Reference Laboratory, a diagnostic facility that specializes in testing for autoimmune diseases, in more than 95% of cases, a negative ANA means that systemic lupus erythematosus (SLE) is not present.

Irritable Bowel Syndrome: Undetected Causes

Medicine has a tendency to define syndromes or conditions, and then treat symptoms but not the cause. This article about irritable bowel syndrome is an example.

ᔷ ᔷ ᔷ

If you are suffering from abdominal cramps, diarrhea, constipation, fatigue, back pain, acne, or allergy symptoms, you could be suffering from irritable bowel syndrome (IBS). IBS is a gastrointestinal disorder that can exist for many years. Treatment is usually directed at symptoms, rather than the cause. This means the symptoms are covered up and a patient is given only temporary relief. In such cases, the underlying cause continues to exist, and the immune system becomes weaker, often leading to more chronic illness.

To correct IBS, one must determine the underlying causes. From my clinical experience, some of the most common causes of IBS are unrecognized food allergies, undetected parasites, and stress. Some questions then arise: Why aren't these causes being investigated? How can one determine the specific causes for one's own situation?

Standard medical training does not address parasites or food allergies as possible causes of IBS. The few standard tests that are available for these conditions have a limited scope for determining a chronic parasite infection or detecting hidden food allergies.

Undiagnosed parasite infections are one of the most neglected problems in the United States. These may account for a great deal of the unexplained causes of IBS. Diagnosis of a parasite infection through a stool sample that may contain ova (eggs) or adult parasites is not a reliable test, unless one has an acute parasite infection. Parasites tend to reside in the intestine, but can travel to the blood, lymph, heart, liver, gallbladder, pancreas, spleen, and brain.

Parasites can produce numerous symptoms, such as abdominal cramps, bloating, weight loss, diarrhea or constipation, allergies, anemia, and immune system disruption. These are all symptoms that are often misdiagnosed as IBS. When hidden parasites are the true cause of symptoms, it means that the wrong treatments will be given and a chronic condition will persist.

For food allergies, I have found the IgG blood tests to be the most reliable tests for detecting a delayed hypersensitivity to foods. One hundred of the most common foods from a typical American diet are tested. Foods that produce the most allergic reactions are often the ones that people consume most frequently: wheat, milk and dairy products, corn, eggs, citrus products, soy, and peanuts.

The following patient story is very typical of a patient with irritable bowel syndrome:

A 31-year-old female came to see me after more than 10 years of suffering with IBS. We conducted food allergy tests and a variety of other diagnostic tests that I commonly use to determine if a chronic parasite problem exists. After eliminating extremely allergic foods and eradicating the parasite infection, the patient became symptom free within a short period of time.

The Truth About Antiaging and Hormone Replacement Therapy

Although many of the benefits of hormone replacement therapy (HRT) have been exaggerated, natural, bioidentical hormones that are well monitored by a physician can deliver a few of the promises. This article provides aging baby boomers with information so they won't fall into traps set by companies that are sizing up the country's second-largest generation. Note: Seventy-six million American babies were born between 1946 and 1960, making the baby boom gencration the nation's second-largest generation. The millennials, (or generation Y) were born from 1978 to 1989. Generation Y is a slightly more populous age group than the baby boomers, making "Y" the largest generation.

૨ઢ ૨ઢ ૨ઢ

Generations of baby boomers are facing the reality of becoming a generation of senior citizens. The last decade has been a quest for the "Holy Grail" of longevity and good health, leading to a new phenomenon of antiaging medicine and hormone replacement therapy.

"Hormone replacement therapy" (HRT) and "antiaging medicine" have become catchphrases meant to attract aging baby boomers with promises of restored vitality, sexuality, and health through an individualized hormone therapy program. If you are a middle-aged woman or man considering the use of HRT, you will be bombarded with hype and confusion. Women are told estrogen will not only protect bones and the heart, but they are also told that hormones will make you feel younger and sexier. They are also told that hormones will stop many menopausal symptoms, such as hot flashes and mood swings. Men are told that testosterone will restore sexual performance and provide youthful vitality and vigor.

The Women's Health Initiative (WHI) study, conducted by the U.S. government's National Institutes of Health (NIH), has shown that synthetic estrogen and progesterone do not protect women from heart disease and osteoporosis. The study also showed that estrogen significantly increases the incidence of breast cancer, uterine cancer, life-threatening blood clots, and Alzheimer's disease.

Conventional HRT relies on synthetic hormones, such as premarin and progestin, which have significant side effects, compared to natural, bioidentical estrogen and progesterone. Ovaries produce 3 different estrogens: estradiol, estrone, and estriol. Ovaries also produce progesterone, testosterone, and DHEA (*and not premarin or progestin*).

What treatment should be given to a woman with menopausal symptoms? Every woman's profile is unique, and treatment must be individualized according to a science-based diagnostic evaluation. Hormone levels of estrogen, progesterone, testosterone, and DHEA can be obtained through blood, saliva, or urine, depending on your doctor's experience.

I believe HRT, even if the hormone is natural and bioidentical, should be used as a last resort and should not be used as the first-line treatment for menopausal symptoms.

The secret of antiaging starts with changes in our consciousness. Longevity comes with healthy living, not just from hormone therapy. One should live an active, full life and grow old gracefully.

The following steps are a good start for healthy living:

Step 1: Water is truly the fountain of life. Drink more water. An average amount is eight 8-ounce glasses of water per day. Spring water is best; filtered tap water is recommended.

Step 2: You are what you eat. Nourish your body with whole foods. A specific nutritional program should be individualized and based on metabolic type, blood type, and food allergies. Food allergies are one of the most overlooked causes of numerous symptoms.

Step 3: You are what you assimilate. Ensure longevity and healthy living by taking digestive enzymes. Enzyme therapy is based upon your diet, metabolism, and the body's acid-base balance.

Step 4: Avoid bad habits. Stop all use of sugar, soda, diet soda, and cigarettes. Smoking and sugar accelerate the aging process.

Step 5: Learn how to cleanse your body using herbal cleansers, fasting, coffee enemas, or colonics.

Step 6: Exercise in moderation. Healing comes when your body is in motion.

Step 7: Control stress at all levels: spiritual, emotional, financial, and physical. Avoid dead-end situations.

Step 8: Remove heavy metals, i.e., mercury, copper, cadmium, lead, and nickel (See: "Our Toxic Planet" in Chapter 4 and "Understanding the Toxins That Get Trapped in Your Liver Ducts" in Chapter 6). Heavy-metal toxicity is an extremely overlooked cause of symptoms. Chelation therapy has been proven to remove heavy-metal toxicity, restore enzyme and immune system function, as well as hormonal balance.

Step 9: And, finally, hormone replacement therapy. HRT should be natural, bioidentical, individualized, and closely monitored by a physician. Appropriate HRT can improve the quality of your life.

These are small steps for restoring your vitality and vigor. HRT is one of the last, but certainly important, steps to take. HRT and anti-aging medicine are catchphrases of the day that may also have misleading information attached. With knowledge, baby boomers can make informed decisions and not be exploited.

Fowl Play on Swine Flu: Medical Marshall Law on Flying Pigs

Busy people who don't have time to read the news media's reports about swine flu may have missed some of the absurd content that is considered to be news. This article will provide samples of a few official stories that were meant to be serious, but sound comical. Because the media reports are so goofy, I've decided to include "Flying Pigs" in my title (*due to the fact that flu officials keep changing their story about the continent where the "swine flu" first appeared*).

🐷 🐷 🐷

In June 2009, soon after a major swine flu outbreak at the flu's epicenter in Mexico, the World Health Organization (WHO) declared that swine flu had reached "pandemic level 6."

To understand this story, it's helpful to realize that the name of the flu has been changed from "swine flu" to "novel H1N1 influenza" to "pandemic H1N1/09 virus," and that the pandemic H1N1/09 virus is a virus containing combinations of avian bird flu, swine flu, and human seasonal influenza flu genetics.

Could it be that a council of pork producers called "foul" for giving this flu the wrong name? Was the sole name "swine flu" a threat to bacon and pork chop sales because it could potentially frighten customers who buy pork products? I'm not sure if this is a joke or not, but it creates an interesting story that explains the flu's name change. I'm glad it's not called Frankenstein flu.

What about the pandemic level 6? What does the WHO and the Centers for Disease Control (CDC) mean when they "raise an alert" to a level 6 pandemic? It means that once a so-called *unstoppable* pandemic level 6 emergency is declared, the WHO can impose regulations, including "quarantine" and other procedures designed to prevent an international spread of the disease. The WHO has the authority to order forced vaccinations around the world under Article 21 of the International Health Regulations (IHR), which was revised in 2005.

It seems that only a few years ago, the WHO was warning us about an impending pandemic avian bird flu similar to the 1918 avian bird flu that took over 20 million lives around the world. The WHO and CDC have been warning us of impending pandemics as they push for vaccinations.

The pandemic avian flu did not materialize, and the public response was less than enthusiastic. As a result, big pharma had lots of left over vaccines at the end of the avian flu season and devised a scare tactic on a gullible public to boost sales of their avian flu vaccine. I have been itching to write an article called "Foul Play on Avian Flu." I was able to change the title to "Fowl Play on Swine Flu."

Over 1 million Americans were exposed to the so-called pandemic H1N1 flu during the summer of 2009. The mortality has been well below 1% (0.06% estimated) in the infected populations, and most of the victims who died were already compromised with preexisting medical conditions.

There is also some concern over the flu vaccination for its safety and also for its effectiveness. What are the ingredients in the flu shot? Most flu shots contain egg proteins, formaldehyde, Triton X100, a detergent, thimerosal, ethyl mercury in multidose vials, polysorbate 80 that can cause severe allergic reactions, squalene used as a vaccine adjuvant that can trigger autoimmune disease, as well as other ingredients. Note: An adjuvant is an agent that is supposed to stimulate the immune system and increase the response to a vaccine, but the truth is adjuvants have been shown to be biological time bombs that harm the immune system.

Knowing the truth about vaccine ingredients means that people with a history of egg allergies, a previous bad reaction to vaccines, or a history of autoimmune disease should avoid a vaccination.

Does the flu shot prevent the flu? Despite CDC claims that the flu vaccination is safe and effective, evidence proves otherwise. Here are statistics that describe the flu vaccine's effectiveness from the Cochrane Database of Systemic Reviews:

- **Children Over 2 Years**
  In children over 2 years, it is only effective 33 percent of the time in preventing the flu.

- **Healthy Adults**
  Vaccination of healthy adults only reduces the risk of influenza by 6 percent and reduces the number of missed work days by less than one (0.16) days.

- **Elderly**
  For the elderly, vaccines are not significantly effective against influenza or pneumonia.

The Department of Homeland Security was the government department chosen to issue this warning to health care providers:

> *The Department of Justice has established legal federal authorities pertaining to the implementation of a quarantine and enforcement.*

To me, it sounds very much like medical Marshall Law on flying pigs and swine flu. Dr. Sherri Tenpenny, D.O., and Dr. Russell Blaylock, M.D., are 2 high-profile doctors in the alternative medical community who are issuing warnings on the misinformation surrounding the pandemic H1N1 and the dangers of the vaccinations. A Google search on either of their names will yield many articles that will help shed light on this very important subject.

I am against mandatory vaccination for swine, avian, seasonal influenza or the pandemic H1N1 flu for the general public. I have received all required vaccinations while I was in the military. Now that I am retired from the military, after 25 years in the Army Reserve, I believe I have a personal choice. I believe the flu vaccination should be a personal choice. Despite predictions of massive numbers of deaths and the arrival of a doomsday, the pandemic H1N1 virus has remained a relatively mild disease like the seasonal influenza flu.

Do not be frightened by jumpy flying pigs and the newest, latest flu. You have a choice whether you want to receive the flu vaccination. If you decide to take a flu vaccine, I hope it does what it's supposed to do and that it protects you from the pandemic H1N1 flu virus. Alternatives that support your immune system include proper nutrition, rest, and avoiding crowded areas.

If you choose to support your immune system, I recommend high potency multivitamins with extra Vitamin C (3,000 mg/day) and natural Vitamin D3 (5,000 U/day). If you develop flu symptoms or a fever and body ache, you must stay at home (self-quarantine), double or triple your Vitamin C and Vitamin D intake, and hydrate well with water until your symptoms subside. A hospital visit is rarely indicated. Chicken soup is a personal option, depending on who makes it.

New Research Indicates Flu Deaths in 1918 Were Due to Overdoses of Aspirin Recommended by Government

In a November 2009 paper, published in the scientific journal called *Clinical Infectious Diseases*, Dr. Karen M. Starko explains that the 1918-1919 influenza pandemic resulted in a high death toll due to extremely "wet," hemorrhagic lungs caused by overdoses of aspirin. Dr. Starko explains that in 1918, the U.S. Surgeon General, the U.S. Navy, and the *Journal of the American Medical Association* recommended use of aspirin just before the October death spike and that physicians during that time were unaware that high doses of aspirin produce levels of hemorrhagic lungs associated with hyperventilation and pulmonary edema.

19

More Crock Pot Ideas

*In questions of science, the authority of
a thousand is not worth the humble
reasoning of a single individual.*
- Galileo Galilei
*Italian physicist, mathematician,
astronomer, and philosopher*

Readers may realize by now that my expression, "crock pot ideas," should not be taken at face value. It's my tongue-in-cheek way of speaking about controversial topics. Fortunately, several men of stature have provided the following advice about telling the truth:

Truth can stand by itself.
- Thomas Jefferson

When in doubt, tell the truth.
- Mark Twain

Speak the truth.
- Confucius

In this chapter, you'll find more of my "crock pot ideas" that were published in *The Healthy Planet* magazine.

Desperate Medicine for Desperate Patients

A November 2009 article that attacked homeopathy prompted me to write this article.

ぞ▲ ぞ▲ ぞ▲

Desperation seems to be the best word to describe the state of medical care in the United States. There is a desperation for a new medical model, but it's not for the proposals in President Obama's Universal Health Care plan.

President Obama's health care plan is based on the same old medical business model with an added twist of politically correct socialized medicine. It does not challenge the shortfall of the current paradigm of pharmacology-dominant medical care and the super-specialization of medicine.

At the same time that this universal health care model is being proposed, there is a strong undercurrent of fear and distrust of current medical care by the public, except for the area of trauma-related emergency care. There is a new tsunami of health care reform arriving, not by politically oriented health care, but by a grassroots movement toward more natural, holistic, integrated medical care. You may call it *desperate medicine for desperate patients*.

As of 2005, cancer became the leading cause of death in this country, surpassing heart disease for the under-85-year-old age group (as per an American Cancer Society report). Cancer and heart disease used to be a rare occurrence 100 years ago. What happened? According to the *Journal of the American Medical Association* (*JAMA*. July 2000; 284), medical care itself (that is, hospital errors and drugs prescribed "properly") is the third leading cause of death.

Patients are afraid to take medications prescribed by their medical doctors. They're also afraid of going to the hospital, unless it is for emergency medical care. People want to know why they are feeling sick, and they want to know how they can prevent illness and stay healthy.

In November 2009, the *American Journal of Medicine* published a commentary on alternative medicine and homeopathy in an article titled, "Should we maintain an open mind about homeopathy?" Written by London-based medical doctors, Michael Baum and Edzard Ernst, the authors say:

> *Homeopathy is among the worst examples of faith-based medicine that gathers shrill support of celebrities and other powerful lobbies in place of a genuine and humble wish to explore the limits of our knowledge using the scientific method.*

In their opinion, if homeopathy is correct, much of physics, chemistry, and pharmacology must be incorrect. They write:

> *A belief in homeopathy exceeds the tolerance of an open mind.*

In the article's conclusion, they write:

> *...it is considered unethical for modern medical practitioners to sink to this kind of deception that denies the patient his or her autonomy. Secondly, by opening the door to irrational medicine alongside evidence-based medicine, we are poisoning the minds of the public.*

Dr. Amy Lansky, Ph.D., author of the best-selling patient education book on homeopathy, wrote a rebuttal to the Baum and Ernst attack on homeopathy (See: "Best-selling Author Explains Why Homeopathy is a Threat to Allopathic Medicine").

Around the same time that the Baum/Ernst article was published, one of the world's largest alternative/complementary medical conferences was being held in Baden Baden, Germany. The conference is called "Medicine Week," and the Germans refer to it as a "European Biological Medicine Congress." Homeopathy, developed by a German medical doctor named Samuel Hahncmann, is very familiar to those who attended the conference. Baum's and Ernst's attempt to disparage Hahnemann's discovery has little effect on the opinions of alternative medical practitioners worldwide who enthusiastically accept the principles of homeopathy.

I was invited to give a lecture at Medicine Week. The title of my lecture was, "Think Parasites When the Latest Medical Therapy Failed: Paradise Lost in the Parallel Universe" (look for a short synopsis of this lecture on my Web site). I was delighted to meet attendees who came from Israel, Turkey, Australia, the Philippines, Canada, the United States, Europe, and many other countries.

One of the difficult questions posed to me has been: "How can you treat for parasites when lab tests are not reliable?" Several members of the audience wanted to know if there is an alternative way to detect parasites. If you have read this far in my book, you already know the answer to this question.

Readers also know about the violin metaphor I've used to help patients understand my energy medicine technique used to diagnose parasites and hidden dental infections. In previous chapters, I have compared an out-of-tune violin to the human body that has out-of-tune energy meridians.

Interestingly, the harmonics of what is considered to be the world's most perfect violin were described in the November 23, 2009 edition of *Time* Magazine. According to this issue, an audience of experts recently took part in a blind test of 5 violins. One of the violins was a 2 million dollar Stradivarius, made in 1711 by the greatest violin maker of all time. Another was a modern violin made of wood that had been specially treated by Professor Francis Schwarze of the Swiss Federal Laboratory for Materials Testing Research. Schwarze used two fungi to alter Norwegian spruce and sycamore to closely resemble the woods Stradivarius used. He then commissioned a violin maker to build an instrument with the treated wood. According to *Time* Magazine, listeners were asked to identify the Stradivarius, and 113 picked Schwarze's violin. The actual Stradivarius received only 39 votes.

In Chapter 3, I compared the EAV device that is used for Acupuncture Meridian Assessment to the strings on a violin—both produce sound. The vibrations of the strings on the violin are transferred to the body of the violin and the sound radiates into the air. The subtle vibrational energy measured at acupoints on the body is also transferred to the EAV device that produces sounds.

It is really not the strings or the acupoints themselves that produce sound, but the interaction with other components. The sound of a violin is the result of a violinist drawing a bow across the strings, causing them to vibrate. This vibration is transmitted to the body of the violin, which increases the loudness of the sound when the energy of the string passes to the face and back plates of the violin. Similarly, the vibrations in a patient's meridians are transferred to the EAV device when a physician touches a probe on acupoints for an Acupuncture Meridian Assessment. The interaction between several components—including a violinist who draws a bow across a string and a physician who presses a probe on an acupoint—is what led me to compare a human body that is sick to a violin that is out of tune. A doctor helps produce sounds that emanate from the EAV device, and he is also the person who does the tuning.

In 2008, Dutch researchers, who published a study in the *Public Library of Science ONE,* said they discovered uniformly dense wood in 5 Stradivarius violins when they passed the instruments through a computed tomography (CT) scanner. The article explains that it is the exceptionally uniform density in the wood that affects the wood's harmonic qualities. It may have been the fungi's effect on the Norwegian spruce and sycamore that altered the wood's grain.

Resonance is a common thread that runs through almost every branch of physics, yet it is not totally understood. The Baum/Ernst attack on the unexplained mysteries of homeopathy is as absurd as an attack on the harmonic perfection of a Stradivarius violin (*or the modern violin made from fungi-treated wood!*).

The evidence-based medicine model described by doctors Baum and Ernst is in crisis. By attacking homeopathy and other alternative medicine therapies, their attitude only perpetuates the shortcomings of traditional medicine. Incidentally, many scientists and physicists take homeopathic remedies themselves because *homeopathy is based on science, physics, and subtle energy.* The Baum/Ernst statements are based on personal biased opinion, and *not* science.

As a conventionally trained medical doctor who has been practicing alternative medicine for the last 20 years, it might be heresy for me to say this:

> *Conventional medical care is like the Stradivarius violin. It's the most expensive, but it doesn't deliver the best medical care.*

We are living in a desperate time with desperate patients looking for desperate medicine. The time to create real change in health care reform, which actually results in healing for patients, is now.

Best-selling Author Explains Why Homeopathy Is a Threat to Allopathic Medicine

The Baum/Ernst article that attacked homeopathy (November 2009, the *American Journal of Medicine*) prompted Dr. Amy Lansky to write a rebuttal that Dr. Joseph Mercola posted on his Web site (www.mercola. com). Lansky was a computer scientist in Silicon Valley when her life was transformed by a homeopathic cure of her 3-year-old son's autism. Her son is now 18, autism free, and a freshman at a leading university. The experience led Amy to write a best-selling book called *Impossible Cure: The Promise of Homeopathy*.

In an article titled, "Why skeptics love to hate homeopathy," published on December 9, 2009, Lansky explains that detractors have succeeded in crippling homeopathic hospitals and clinics in the United Kingdom, even though Prince Charles and the rest of the royal family are ardent supporters of homeopathic medicine.

Amy's article also helps readers to understand that homeopathy has been one of the most threatening alternative modalities since the 1800s. The history she provides explains that Hahnemann was forced to move frequently because the local German apothecaries objected to the fact that he created his own medicine. She describes homeopathy's strong presence in the United States, and the battle that was waged against homeopathic remedies that were successfully used in the treatment of cholera, typhus, yellow fever, diphtheria, influenza, and other epidemics of the 1800s. The American Medical Association (AMA) was formed in 1847—specifically to fight homeopathy. The AMA charter forbade AMA members to associate with homeopaths.

The biggest reason that homeopathy is a threat to allopathic medicine is due to the method used to prepare homeopathic remedies. Hahnemann discovered that ultradilutions of homeopathic remedies were even more potent than stronger dilutions. These ultradilutions were so dilute, they did not contain a single molecule of the original substance.

Since Hahnemann's discovery of the potency of ultradilutions, there have been several scientific studies indicating that an energy signature of the original substance is embedded in the ultradilution. The biggest reason why big pharma has contempt for homeopathy is due to the:

ultradilutions

Poor countries, such as India and Cuba, have already discovered ultradilutions, and they're using them successfully.

The only rub in homeopathic medicine is that there are no cookie-cutter cures. (I have already explained this to my readers.) Because each patient is unique, a homeopath must treat each patient individually. It may take a homeopath several tries to find the right remedy among thousands of possible homeopathic remedies.

Today, Lansky is an executive board member of the National Center for Homeopathy (www.nationalcenterforhomeopathy.org) and hosts a monthly radio show on Autism One Radio (autismone.org).

Location, Location, Location: Geopathic Disturbance Causes Sickness

Readers will be surprised to learn that German physicians who study biological medicine routinely check their patients for illnesses caused by geopathic disturbance, which is rarely investigated in the United States. My article on geopathic disturbance provides an introduction to this unfamiliar but important topic.

ॐ ॐ ॐ

I'm not talking about the golden rule of real estate when I say location, location, location. I'm talking about a faulty bed arrangement in your bedroom due to geopathic disturbances that affect your health. If your bed is in a zone of geopathic disturbance, you may develop many unexplained medical symptoms, as well as an unsuspected illness while you're sleeping.

There are many theories and names for geopathic disturbance. It is more commonly called "earth radiation" or "earth rays." Other names include "Curry lines" (named after Manfred Curry, M.D.), "earth faults," and "cosmic energy shadows." Earth rays emit radiation from the earth above subterranean water currents. The disturbances created by these earth rays are called geopathic zones.

Some people are highly sensitive to earth rays—both physically and emotionally. This sensitivity is called "radiesthesia." These individuals tend to be thin, fair skinned, serious minded, altruistic, highly sensitive, easily hurt, and they are often young children. I have been studying German biological medicine for 15 years, and I have learned that German practitioners are very aware of geopathic disturbances.

It usually takes months or even years for the body to become sensitized and weakened from geopathic radiation. Bacteria and parasites thrive in geopathic energy and can easily infect people who are already weakened from sleeping in a radiated area. These invaders are also more likely to multiply rapidly in a weakened immune system of someone who is sensitive to these zones. How do you know if you're affected by geopathic disturbances or earth rays?

Those affected by these disturbances have often seen numerous medical doctors and alternative practitioners without success. In my practice, I address common medical problems that are often overlooked by traditional medical doctors, and I have learned to consider geopathic disturbances when all else fails.

My list of common medical problems, which I have reviewed several times in this book include:

- Heavy-metal toxicity
- Food allergies
- Hidden infections, including parasites
- Nutritional deficiencies
- Unsuspected dental-related medical problems

The majority of my patients respond and feel better when most of these major underlying problems are corrected. However, not every patient responds, and occasionally I have a patient who has unusual, persistent symptoms or who suffers from recurrent infections.

When all else fails, consider that geopathic disturbances might be the cause of your unsuspected illness. In her book, *Discoveries of a Dowser*, Austrian researcher Käthe Bachler lists the following ten indicators that a pathogenic zone of disturbance may be present in the bedroom:

- Aversion to going to bed (especially in children)
- Not being able to go to sleep for hours (insomnia)
- Restless sleep, crumpled-up sheets, nightmares, falling out of bed, and crying out

- Avoidance of certain spots in a bed, as well as rocking and head banging
- Sleepwalking
- Feeling cold, as well as shivering, grinding teeth, and night sweats in bed
- Fatigue and apathy in the morning that lasts through the day
- Lack of appetite, which may include vomiting in the morning
- Despondency, nervousness, depression, and "just not feeling well"
- Cramps, and/or increased heart rate in bed

According to Vienna's Dr. Hilde Plenk, any one of these symptoms should be considered to be a clue that a geopathic disturbance exists—especially after exhaustive tests.

In a paper titled, "Observations from a Geobiological Practice" (1975), German medical doctor, Dieter Achoff, M.D., reported that he had achieved astounding results in his medical practice by relocating his patients' beds. He wrote:

> *No longer does a physician need great courage to discuss these facts with his patients, since the phenomena now enjoy general knowledge, due to all the experiments that have been conducted over the years. The physician who is cognizant of the existence of zones of disturbance can turn the wheel of destiny to his patients' advantage.*

Once you are aware of geopathic disturbance as a possibility for an unexplained illness in your family, the question becomes, "So, what do I do now?" Bächler, Achoff, and other researchers recommend rearranging a bed and observing the results. In her book, Bächler explains that she discovered geopathic energy when she moved her asthmatic son's bed. His asthma disappeared, and she kept searching for answers to what appeared to be an unexplained mystery. Bächler sought the help of a well-respected dowsers group in Vienna. Members in the group taught her how to dowse. After dowsing over 4,000 homes, she wrote her book. To investigate the energy in your home:

- Follow your intuition. Rearrange your bed and observe the results, as Bächler did when her son suffered from asthma.

- Seek the assistance of an experienced, professional dowser who can help locate geopathic energy with dowsing tools. You may do a Google search for "Dowser in Saint Louis, Missouri" or the location where you live, and have the selected person dowse your home or place of work.

Animals can help locate geopathic energy due to their sensitive instincts. Readers with dogs or cats can follow their pets' instincts by paying attention to the following rules:

- Dogs avoid earth rays. Even an obedient dog will not heed his master's command if ordered to lie on a radiated spot. Find a spot where dogs like to sleep in the bedroom and that can be the spot for your bed.

What Is Dowsing?

Dowsing is the practice "of locating something by using sensory means other than the 5 senses of sight, sound, taste, touch, and smell." A dowser's tools include a Y-shaped twig, an L-Rod, or a pendulum.

- Horses, cows, pigs, chickens, and birds avoid earth rays.
- As a rule, cats are earth ray seekers. Avoid spots where cats like to sleep in the bedroom.
- Bees, ants, insects, bacteria, and parasites are earth ray seekers.

Be educated and not medicated. Find a location for your bed without geopathic disturbances, and be healthy and happy. In a book titled, *Dowsing Manual*, Australian author and researcher Harald W. Tietze provides the following quote from Michael Nostradamus, the famous French physician and seer, who is known mostly by just his last name "Nostradamus:"

> *Where plants perish and animals are absent, there you also should not live. The place is unhealthy. You will experience disharmony and lose your poise. When you, however, find the place where happy, vital, and healthy people live, and many old folks in good health, then stay there. You soon do without medicine or physicians. The mysterious forces of Earth make you healthy.*

Dr. Semmelweis on Death Due to Childbed Fever

Unrecognized infection's role in chronic illness is described in this article that I wrote about a young Hungarian doctor named Ignaz Semmelweis who helped large numbers of women survive childbirth in the mid-19th century. Although Semmelweis knew nothing about germs, he introduced a strict hand-washing policy for physicians who worked in obstetrical units. More than 150 years later, most medical practitioners are still very much in the dark about microbes and parasites that cause chronic disease. This time, the microbes are not lingering on physicians' hands—they're hiding in the body! My article includes stories about 2 women patients, both unusual cases, who experienced dramatic improvements in their health after taking several prescription antiparasite medications.

꙰ ꙰ ꙰

Ignaz Semmelweis, a young Hungarian doctor working in the obstetrical ward of a Vienna Hospital in the late 1840s, was alarmed at the high death rate among his patients. He had noticed that nearly twenty percent of the women under his and his colleagues' care died shortly after childbirth. The cause of death was identified as "Childbed Fever." He also noticed that the death rate was 4 to 5 times higher than the death rate in a ward attended by female midwives who had no advanced medical training. A breakthrough came in 1847 following the death of Ignaz's good friend, Jakob Kolletschka, who was accidentally poked with a scalpel while performing a postmortem examination. Kolletschka's autopsy showed a pathological abnormality similar to that observed in women who died from childbed fever. Semmelweis immediately proposed a connection between cadaveric contamination and childbed fever.

To salvage the high death rate due to childbed fever in his own ward, Dr. Semmelweiss instituted a strict hand-washing policy for male students and attending physicians when they came from the autopsy room to the delivery room. Believe it or not, at the time, it was a common practice to perform an autopsy, then go directly to an obstetrics ward to deliver babies without hand washing!

Semmelweis' rule required everyone to wash their hands with chlorinated lime water prior to attending patients. Mortality rates immediately dropped from 18.3% to 1.3%. Not a single woman died from childbirth between March and August 1848 in the Semmelweis obstetrical ward. Despite the dramatic reduction in the mortality rate in Semmelweis' ward, his colleagues and the greater medical community in Vienna greeted his finding with hostility and contempt. This occurred, even when he presented his finding to the Viennese Medical Society.

After years of controversy and repeated rejection of his work by the medical community, Semmelweis suffered a mental breakdown. He died in 1865 in an Austrian mental institution.

Semmelweiss' story reminds me of 2 patients named Rose and Kelly. When I met Rose, an 86-year-old widow with 6 children, she had kidney cancer that had spread to her lung. Rose's prognosis was grim—she had been given 3 months to live. Surprisingly, chemotherapy had been recommended, even though she was told that she would die in a few months. Rose did not like the options that had been presented to her. She wanted a second opinion. She came to see me with 2 of her adult children. One of Rose's children was open to alternative medicine, and the other was almost hostile to any form of integrative medicine.

My evaluation of Rose started with an Acupuncture Meridian Assessment that is described in several sections in this book. I discovered that Rose's main disturbance signals came from the liver, stomach, pancreas, and large intestine meridians. Her kidney and lung meridians were in fairly good condition, despite her diagnosis

What Does Metastasize Mean?

In a cancer patient, metastasize refers to the spread of cancer cells, causing secondary tumors. The cells in the metastatic tumor are like those in the original cancer.

of kidney cancer that had metastasized to her lung. She started taking antiparasite medications that included alinia, praziquantel, ivermectin, as well as detoxification herbs, homeopathic remedies, and combinations of antioxidants.

Eighteen months later, Rose was as spunky as ever. She had no complaints except for the "hardship" of taking all those vitamins and minerals. I'm not actively following her with computed tomography (CT) scans, but she has no signs of active cancer. I joke with Rose and tell her that I believe that she will outlive her oncologist—and possibly her children.

Kelly, my other patient, whom I remembered when I learned about Semmelweis' story, had breast cancer with a highly unusual pain in her breast. I saw Kelly in September 2007. She was 49 years old at the time and had recently been diagnosed with breast cancer. After a lumpectomy, she developed a burning pain in her left breast, as well as her shoulder blade. Kelly had a history of multiple chemical sensitivities that prompted her to wear wooden shoes and carry her own wooden chair. She could not tolerate any chemicals and rode in a van for 3 hours—on her wooden chair—the day of her visit.

When I met Kelly, her behavior seemed very peculiar, weird, and restless. Her Acupuncture Meridian Assessment indicated multiple meridian disturbances on allergy points, as well as her spleen, kidney, stomach, liver, gallbladder, and pancreas meridians. After her visit, I started her on gentle, homeopathic detoxification remedies.

As Kelly grew stronger, I was able to start her on multiple courses of antiparasite medications, including tinidazole, mebendazole, pyrantel pamoate, alinia, and ivermectin. The last time I saw Kelly in January 2009, she no longer had the unusual pain in her breast. She also appeared calm and happy. In fact, she seemed more concerned about her husband's health than her own.

I treated Rose and Kelly with many different nutritional supplements, homeopathic remedies, and body detoxification herbs. As I've described in this article, they were both given unique antiparasite medications that were specific to their individual evaluation.

Unrecognized infection, caused by bacteria, viruses, fungi, or larger parasitic worms, seem to play a major role in most chronic illnesses. From an evolutionary point of view, microbes and especially larger parasitic worms are very intelligent creatures that have adapted to constant changes in the environment from the beginning of life on Earth. They invade a host and reproduce in a most extraordinary and complex life cycle. These parasitic aliens are constantly invading our bodies, and they play an important role in unexplained, chronic illness.

Semmelweis did not know much about microbes, but he knew handwashing dramatically reduced childbed fever and its death rate in Vienna in the 1840s. I've been prescribing antiparasite medications to balance acupuncture meridians and, in the 15 years that I have been using these drugs, I have noticed that patients with some of the most difficult health problems begin to improve.

The lesson of these stories is not "Don't see the chauvinistic male doctor from Vienna," but to understand why there was such resistance to change. Even if the role of infectious microbes was not understood at the time, overwhelming facts supported the importance of hand washing for the prevention of childbed fever. What were those prominent physicians in Vienna thinking? Why did they dismiss Semmelweis' finding?

I don't fully understand why parasite medications balance so many disturbed meridians, or why these drugs cause difficult illnesses to disappear. There seem to be many infectious microbes, as well as larger, parasitic worms, that are not easily detected by current medical science. We need young scientists to investigate and validate parasite-related phenomena.

There are too many Roses and Kellys, and others who suffer unnecessarily from current medical care. We need to think differently! Rather than rejecting nontraditional thinkers, we need a new generation of men and women like Dr. Semmelweiss to save us from the death trap of the modern scourges of heart disease, cancer, and iatrogenic (doctor-induced) death. I will continue to use antiparasite medications based on my Acupuncture Meridian Assessments until there are better biometric systems that can detect hidden infections.

Do You Have MUS (Multiple Unexplained Symptoms or Syndrome)?

Allopathic medical doctors are slowly being asked to practice "evidence-based medicine" that is based on research published in medical journals. The problem is, published research says that 50 percent of all patients have "unexplained medical symptoms." The article, titled, "Do you have MUS? Is this standard medical care according to the evidence-based medicine model?" explains this conundrum.

≈ ≈ ≈

If you have MUS (medically unexplained symptoms), you are not alone. What exactly is MUS and what are the implications of this mysterious condition?

A report from the Veterans Administration's (VA) War-Related Illness and Injury Study Center of New Jersey, published in September 2009, explains:

Medically unexplained symptoms (MUS) is a term used for health symptoms, which remain unexplained after a complete medical evaluation. It has been reported that vague health symptoms account for half of all outpatient visits and that one third of these symptoms remain unexplained after a thorough assessment (Jackson et al, 2005).

Although common, presence of symptoms which remain unexplained for long periods of time, even after a medical evaluation, can be confusing and frustrating for both patients and providers. Patients who have multiple unexplained symptoms over a period of time may meet the criteria for the diagnosis of a "medically unexplained syndrome (MUS). Being given a diagnosis of MUS can be a relief, although management of these multiple symptoms can be challenging.

I had never heard of MUS as a new diagnosis until I read a major medical journal in 2009. I then started searching for the latest information on MUS. The VA report that I have referenced describes 3 specific MUS conditions: chronic fatigue syndrome (CFS), fibromyalgia (FM), and irritable bowel syndrome (IBS). What's missing in the VA report is a detailed explanation of why "vague health (or MUS) symptoms account for half of all outpatient visits." A clue that may explain this rather startling news is the Jackson et al citation in the VA report (Jackson et al, 2005).

It turns out that the Jackson in the VA citation is Dr. Jeffrey L. Jackson, M.D., an internist with the Department of Defense's (DOD) Department of Medicine, Uniformed Services University of the Health Sciences. Jackson and his colleagues have collaborated on several articles about "unexplained syndromes" over the past 10 years—frequently recommending psychiatric drugs. Examples include:

"Antidepressant therapy for unexplained symptoms and symptom syndromes" *The Journal of Family Practice,* 1999 December; 48:980–90, O'Malley P.G., Jackson J.L., Santoro J., et al.

"Antidepressants and cognitive-behavioral therapy for symptom syndromes" Jackson J.L., O'Malley P.G., Kroenke K., *CNS Spectrums: The International Journal of Neuropsychiatric Medicine,* 2006 March;11(3):212-22. A review.

"Outcome and iImpact of mental disorders in primary care at 5 years," *Psychosomatic Medicine* 69:270–276 (2007), Jeffrey L. Jackson, M.D., MPH, Mark Passamonti, M.D., and Kurt Kroenke, M.D.

In the *Psychosomatic Medicine* article, Dr. Jackson and his coauthors say, "Mental disorders are prevalent in primary care, present in up to a third of patients." They add that mental disorders are "frequently missed" and cite *one* "systematic review" that says that mental disorders have an "overall undiagnosed rate of fifty percent."

Has MUS evolved out of "one systematic review" cited by Dr. Jackson and his cohorts who appear to be aggressively writing articles about "unexplained symptoms" and "symptom syndromes" for the medical literature?

If there are so many patients with MUS, how can one treat MUS patients when the "evidence-based medicine" model taught at medical teaching institutions cannot (or will not) figure out the cause of the problems? (See: "What is Evidence-Based Medicine?")

Are medical students being taught that all unexplained symptoms are "psychosomatic?" I feel sorry for medical students and doctors

What Is Evidence-Based Medicine (EBM)?

The term "Evidence-based medicine" first appeared in the medical literature in 1992 in a paper by Guyatt et al (written by 30 colleagues in The Evidence-Based Medical Working Group). The article is titled, "Evidence-based medicine. A new approach to teaching the practice of medicine," and was published in the *Journal of the American Medical Association* (*JAMA* 268 (17): 2420–5. November 1992). The authors introduce readers to a "new paradigm" for medical practice" that "de-emphasizes intuition, unsystematic clinical experience, and pathophysiological rationale as sufficient grounds for decision making" and stresses the "examination of evidence" from clinical research that is "double-blind" and "randomized."

Note: The pathophysiology that The Evidence-Based Working Group said should be "de-emphasized" is the physiology of abnormal states or the functional changes that accompany a particular syndrome or disease.

Advice that tells physicians to "de-emphasize" changes that accompany disease is at odds with an entire branch of alternative medicine called "functional medicine." Functional medical doctors focus on improving physiological function to improve health. The Institute for Functional Medicine defines this approach as "personalized medicine that deals with primary prevention and underlying causes, instead of symptoms, for serious chronic disease." Functional medical doctors believe that diet, nutrition, and exposure to environmental toxins play central roles in health because they predispose a patient to illness, provoke symptoms, and change the body's biochemistry.

in training. Most MUS patients feel they are out of whack or out of tune, yet no lab test or medical evaluations show abnormalities.

After learning the intricate medical science and rituals of clinical training, medical professionals diagnose numerous chronically ill patients as MUS. Medical professionals then end up treating the symptoms for such illnesses as chronic fatigue syndrome, fibromyalgia, and irritable bowel syndrome with medications that include antidepressants. This is the current standard medical care! Do you think there's any influence from pharmaceutical companies on our medical training?

I wonder what Galileo Galilei would say about current standard medical care based on the evidence-based medicine model. Galileo, the radical contrarian astronomer of his time, said, "In questions of science, the authority of a thousand is not worth the humble reasoning of a single individual." Most people intuitively understand that something is missing in their medical diagnosis and treatment. They feel something is not right, and they know the problems are not in their head.

Evidence-based medicine (EBM) has met MUS! EBM has been losing credibility and the public's trust. It is medicine that is based on measurable and quantifiable science or linear, compartmentalized thinking that leads us to the question, "...if everything has to be double-blinded, randomized, and evidence-based, where does that leave new ideas?" (*The Lancet*, Volume 366, Issue 9480, Pages 122-122, J. Wu, July 9-15, 2005 "Could evidence-based medicine be a danger to progress?").

Some of my fibromyalgia patients respond after correcting their dental cavitations (jaw bone infections), IBS patients respond to antiparasite medications, and chronic fatigue patients respond to combinations of dental work, parasite eradications, and nutritional therapy. Some of my patients with advanced metastatic cancer respond to intensive detoxification, nutritional therapies, and parasite medications. Others find that extraction of asymptomatic root canal teeth relieves palpitations, chest pain, arthritic pain, and asthma.

So, do you have MUS? Evidence-based medicine is not ready to solve the mystery of MUS. I propose a new standard medical care that starts with intestinal parasite cleansing, removal of mercury dental amalgams and hidden dental infections, elimination of foods from one's diet that cause food allergies, initiation of individualized nutritional programs based on blood or tissue mineral analysis, and inclusion of detoxification using a gallbladder/liver flush protocol.

All of the combined therapies that I have mentioned are a good starting point for most MUS patients. In addition, other tangible and intangible variables may need to be part of an individualized health plan including:

- Changes in diet

- Rest

- Sleep

- Stress control

- Detoxification

- Prayer

Oddly, in the eyes of evidence-based medicine, some of the dramatic healing responses to the regimen I've mentioned are referred to as "placebo effects." Healing often occurs from the regimen I have mentioned. However, the healing may seem unpredictable and random to an outside observer who has no prior experience with this form of healing. Confusion exists because healing may not happen instantly and may not occur until a full regimen is utilized over a period of time.

It is sometimes difficult to understand how these therapies may be related to one's current health problems. However, they are all interrelated. Our bodies operate according to biomechanical, biochemical, bioelectrical, and biophysical principles that encompass a unified whole of body/mind/spirit. During the course of these therapies, your body will begin to heal on its own. As you get well, let's call it an "accidental cure."

Today's Medical Journal Articles and Family Medicine Curriculum—for Young Doctors— Reflect Information Technology Trends

In 1990, the *Journal of the American Medical Association* called medical informatics "an emerging academic discipline and institutional priority." Medical informatics (or computerized medicine) has been called the "intersection of information science, computer science, and health care."

Young doctors are being taught to integrate a computer in their relationship with patients. A curriculum guideline titled, "Recommended Curriculum Guidelines for Family Medicine Residents," endorsed by the American Academy of Family Physicians, says:

> *Didactic lectures (textbook and lecture instruction) should be augmented with instruction regarding principles of the doctor-patient-computer relationship in daily practice.*

Young doctors are also being steered away from an "individual" model to a "population-based" model through technology applications.

The same curriculum-guideline document says a resident in family medicine should demonstrate the ability to apply knowledge of:

- *Basic components of computer systems, networks, and the nature of computer-human interfaces as they impact patient care.*

- *Fundamentals of data modeling and database systems (including the definition and application of controlled vocabularies and structured versus unstructured data types).*

- *Application of aggregation and analysis of clinical data for improving care quality and patient outcomes.*

With the addition of a computer in the "doctor-patient" relationship and all the databasing that's being added to conventional medicine, it may be hard for a young doctor to choose an alternative medicine track and wrestle free from allopathic medicine's emphasis on "population studies," rather than a study of the "individual."

Since The Evidence-Based Medical Working Group wrote their 1992 paper (See: What is Evidence-Based Medicine [EBM]?"), medical journals have published studies about clinical trials with several new types of biomedical research experiment designs and information management (See: "Today's Medical Journal Articles and Family Medicine Curriculum—for Young Doctors—Reflect Information Technology Trends"). Computerized medicine and the pressure to practice "evidence-based medicine" push doctors to evaluate patients with statistics and leave no

room for physicians' clinical experience with patients.
Evidence-based medicine completely ignores:

- Physicians' skills that evaluate patients as a whole

- The importance of history taking, the physical
  examination, and classical methods of patient evaluation

- Analytical and critical diagnostic thinking

- The skills of etiologic and differential diagnosis
  (Etiological diagnosis refers to a search for the cause
  or origin of a disease)

No wonder *The Lancet*, the world's most prestigious
medical journal founded in 1823, published an article in
2005 titled, "Could evidence-based medicine be a danger
to progress?"

Part 6

Conclusion

We can't solve problems by using the same kind of thinking we used when we created them.

The most incomprehensible thing about the world is that it is comprehensible.

- Albert Einstein

Notes

20

Time to Heal: New Medicine Based on New Biology

Time is the coin of your life. It is the only coin you have, and only you can determine how it will be spent. Be careful lest you let other people spend it for you.
- Carl Sandburg
American Poet

After unsuccessful chemotherapy and radiation therapy, advanced cancer patients often come to see me for a cure as a last resort. At the end of the session, we often end up talking about time.

The patient usually asks me "How much time do I have? Is there any hope for a cure?" My typical response is "I don't know." I will dodge the questions with vague explanations because there are far too many variables in life, including fate and God's will.

So, what is time? I want you to relax. I am not going to bore you with Einstein's theory of relativity, global scaling mathematics, New Age metaphysics, or mind-bending fractals. What matters is our perception of time.

The Story of the Bank Account Makes You Think About Time

While I was reviewing some of my old conference lecture materials, I found a story about "time." Time affects every aspect of life as soon as we wake up in our own unique *time scale*. This story, called "The Bank Account," makes you think about the value of every second of every day:

> Imagine there is a bank that credits your account each morning with $86,400 (there are 86,400 seconds per day). It carries over no balance from day to day. Every evening it deletes whatever part of the balance you failed to use during the day. What would you do? Draw out every cent, of course.

> Each of us has such a bank. Its name is TIME. Every morning it credits you with 86,400 seconds for the day. Every night it writes off, as lost, whatever of this you have failed to invest to a good purpose. It carries over no balance. It shows no overdraft. Each day it opens a new account for you. Each night it burns the remains of the day. If you fail to use the day's deposits, the loss is yours. There is no going back. There is no drawing against the "tomorrow."

> You must live in the present on today's deposits. Invest it so as to get from it the utmost in health, happiness, and success. The clock is running. Make the most of today.

> *To realize the value of One Year, ask a student who has failed a grade.*

> *To realize the value of One Month, ask a mother who has given birth to a premature baby.*

> *To realize the value of One Week, ask an editor of a weekly newspaper.*

> *To realize the value of One Day, ask a daily wage laborer who has kids to feed.*

> *To realize the value of One Hour, ask the lovers who are waiting to meet.*

> *To realize the value of One Minute, ask a person who has missed the train.*

To realize the value of One Second, ask a person who has avoided an accident.

To realize the value of One Millisecond, ask the person who has won a silver medal in the Olympics.

Treasure every moment that you have! And treasure it more because you shared it with someone special; special enough to have your time…and remember time waits for no one. Yesterday is history; tomorrow, a mystery. Today is a gift; that's why it's called the present!

Each individual has a different meaning for "time." While you are reading this chapter, it may resonate or move your heart differently—based on your life experience. For me, I can feel my heart start to quibble when I read the line, "To realize the value of One Day, ask a daily wage laborer who has kids to feed." What about you?

It Takes Time to Correct Underlying Problems

Every chronic illness has multiple causes. It takes time to correct underlying problems, and the goal is to correct as many as possible. With enough time, one's body will heal itself of most minor illnesses. Time is the best healer. The "time to heal" or the healing time is an unknown. We have our own unique *time scale* for healing.

When an advanced cancer patient or ALS (amyotrophic lateral sclerosis or Lou Gehrig's disease) patient comes to see me for an evaluation, the patient and I understand that we are racing against time to beat the odds of the inevitable—dying and death. So, where do we start?

The patient's life history, including a medical history (past), takes us to the current situation (present), and gives us a glimpse of the future outcome (tomorrow). Most people do not recognize the seemingly unrelated and underlying chain of events that lead into the present medical condition—and how it affects their future medical outcome.

For My Patient Jane, Healing Time Was Short

Recently, I saw Jane, a young mother with severe irritable bowel syndrome (IBS), including typical symptoms of diarrhea and abdominal cramps. She was on multiple medications and had been in and out of the hospital (a place that she desperately wanted to avoid).

Jane's story starts as a young girl who had frequent ear infections (she probably had food allergies), and had grown up taking multiple antibiotics. In her early twenties, Jane had several root canals and later suffered from constant sinus congestion, sinus infections, as well as bronchial infections that were frequently treated with antibiotics.

During a recent ear infection, Jane tried several different antibiotics and later developed her diarrhea and abdominal cramps, in addition to a whole list of other unexplained physical symptoms.

When Jane came to see me, her evaluation included an Acupuncture Meridian Assessment. I started her on probiotics and antiparasite medications. Within a few days, Jane's bowel movements stabilized, her abdominal cramps subsided, and she was able to stay out of the hospital.

For My Patient Laura, Time Was Critical

In August 2008, I saw Laura, a 43-year-old woman from Iowa, who was going blind due to a suspected amoeba infection. Laura had been evaluated by numerous ophthalmologists at a teaching hospital in Iowa and was not responding to antiparasitic medications. Her doctors suspected that her infection may have been due to her contact lenses.

Because Laura was not responding to medications, she was told to apply for Social Security disability for blindness. Laura, like many desperate patients, was looking to and willing to try any therapy — conventional or alternative — to slow down the loss of her eyesight.

I saw Laura as an emergency case the next day after she was informed about her situation. According to her Acupuncture Meridian Assessment, she had disturbances in her liver, gallbladder, and stomach meridians. Even though Laura had been given antiparasite medications, the drugs or the dosage were either incorrect, or they were given in the wrong combination. I started her on triple parasite medications including mebendazole, tinidazole, and alinia. She was instructed to repeat the medications in 2 weeks.

Within a few weeks, there was a dramatic improvement in Laura's eyesight with no sign of amoeba activity in her eyes. At a follow-up visit, her gallbladder, liver, and stomach meridians were normal and so was her vision. Laura has not come back for any further follow-up visits. I was told she has been doing well, her eyesight has been totally restored, and she has not applied for disability.

Disappearance of Symptoms Does Not Mean the Body Is Cured

Most people assume the disappearance of symptoms means they are cured. However, it will take many months of treatment for the body to reorganize and truly heal itself. Jane and Laura were not interested in any further treatment for financial reasons. Jane was not interested in dental work. In Laura's case, the ophthalmologists from the teaching hospital were not interested in my evaluation, or the treatment for parasites based on new ideas and technology. In fact, she was instructed not to discuss her illness and not to give a testimonial for my book.

Racing against time is essential for people who have far more advanced and life-threatening medical problems than Jane and Laura. Balancing and maintaining the meridians and tuning "the violin" is my job as a physician. Not everyone responds to my therapy. It is up to the individual patient how they practice and play "the violin" in the symphony of life. The symphony of life is timeless. By understanding that healing comes from within and that you are responsible for your own healing, you can change the scale of the *time to heal*.

New Medicine Based on New Biology: Quantum Medicine

Energy medicine is a new buzzword in the field of alternative medicine with a new twist: new medicine based on quantum physics. Is quantum physics' wave-particle duality as relevant in biology as Newtonian mechanistic concepts of universal gravitation force and acceleration or Einstein's theory of relativity in space and time? (See: "Quantum Physics vs. Classical Physics.") A new generation of scientists and biologists think it is.

For these new scientists, traditional biologists and medical scientists— committed a gross scientific error by overlooking quantum physics as being too weird, mind bending, and unpredictable for biological systems. Truthfully, quantum physics *is* mind bending, except that recently, the reality of quantum physics or quantum effects has been simplified by observations in animals and plants. The "new" medicine states that this reality also applies to all living systems.

Plants Employ a Quantum Effect to Capture the Energy of the Sun

In living systems, green plants and certain green bacteria capture energy from the photons of sunlight and use it to make food through photosynthesis. The initial stage of the process is so efficient that scientists are looking at quantum phenomena to explain the efficiency of harvesting photons and efficient electron transport at the atomic level. According to theoretical physicist, Thorsten Ritz, Ph.D., when excited by a photon, chlorophyll molecules no longer act as individuals, but band together to create a system that works in concert.

Migrating Birds Use Quantum Effects to Sense Magnetic Fields

Migrating birds exploit quantum effects in their visual systems to sense magnetic fields. In a 2004 *Nature* study, Thorsten Ritz and his colleagues showed that disrupting the local magnetic field around

Quantum Physics vs. Classical Physics

For those of you who are not familiar with quantum physics, it is an exciting branch of physics that emerged a century ago when classical physics was unable to explain the behavior of very small amounts of matter and small units of light (called photons). The mystery behavior that is still perplexing relates to matter that behaves like particles some of the time (similar to billiard balls) and like waves at other times (similar to water waves). These two behaviors are called quantum physics' wave-particle duality for short.

Very recently, an interesting development has occurred. For a century, quantum effects could only be expressed mathematically because the effects described behavior of very small particles, such as photons and electrons.

Within the last few years, scientists have started to observe quantum effects in nature—in bird behavior and in photosynthesis. Previously, the laws of motion and force have been totally dominated by theories developed by physicists Isaac Newton (1643–1727) and Albert Einstein (1879–1955). Newton's *Principia Mathematica,* published in 1687, is considered to be among the most influential books in the history of science.

In his book, Newton says that everything—from orbiting planets to falling apples and all the large and small phenomena of gravity—are caused by 1 of 2 kinds of forces:

- Pulling force of attraction

- Pushing force of repulsion

In 1916, Einstein advanced Newton's theories of force and motion in what is known as his "theory of relativity." Einstein theorized that a uniform gravitational field (like that near the earth) is equivalent to a uniform acceleration. This means that a person cannot tell the difference between:

- Effect A
  Standing on the earth, feeling the effects of gravity as a downward pull

- Effect B
  Standing in a very smooth elevator that is accelerating upwards at just the right rate of exactly 32 feet per second squared.

Occasionally, Britain's Royal Society (the world's oldest scientific society that was founded in 1662) surveys its members and asks them to name the scientist who had the greatest effect on the history of science—Newton or Einstein. In 1999, Einstein was voted the "greatest physicist ever" and, in 2005, Newton was considered to be the most influential.

The fact that there are only two scientists on the ballot reflects how much physics has been in a holding pattern since Newton wrote his *Principia Mathematica* in 1687.

captive birds preparing to migrate interfered with the birds' internal compasses. The discoveries concerning quantum effects in green plants and birds have fostered the idea that all other living systems have been living in the world of quantum physics. For the past hundred years, *quantum physicists* have been describing the behavior of photons (units of light) and electrons in the *subatomic world.* Now, scientists realize that "quantum" is at life's foundation and that it's a process that's part of a larger biology. This new (and larger) aspect of quantum physics is called *living physics* (Susan Galdos. *Science News.* May 2009.)

Cells Communicate Through Vibrational Frequency

Think of the body as a microcosm of the universe. There are about 100 trillion living cells in each of our bodies; only 10 trillion cells are considered human cells. This smaller number of cells make up the brain, heart, lung, kidney, muscle, liver, pancreas, and other organs. The other 90 trillion cells are foreign, alien cells living in our bodies as bacteria, fungus, viruses, and other advanced complex organisms that exist in symbiotic harmony most of the time. These cells have been sharing DNA information and evolving with us from the time that we were born.

How does communication and the coordination of complex biochemical reactions take place in a body with 10 trillion human cells and 90 trillion foreign cells? Classical biology says this occurs with the help of biochemical pathways, hormones, neuropeptides, and the nervous system. According to professor Fritz A. Popp, Ph.D., a biophysicist—cells, and therefore organs, communicate by vibration frequency in waves and photon particles (See: Professor Fritz A. Popp, Ph.D., in Chapter 2). Every living system seems to be regulated upside down and inside out by quantum physics.

DNA in the Quantum World

In the quantum world, chromosomal DNA operates like a micro-crystal antenna, constantly resonating and transmitting information to multiple targeted genes for multiple genetic expressions that are based on the influence of the environment. Remarkably, cell biologists have discovered that DNA receives information through cell membrane's receptor proteins called integral membrane proteins (IMPs). The cell membrane's importance grew when scientists discovered this function. Previously, it was thought that the cell nucleus controlled the cell because it housed a cell's DNA.

According to Bruce Lipton, Ph.D., in his book, *The Biology of Belief*, the genetic material inside the nucleus is equivalent to a cell's gonad. Lipton calls the cell membrane the cell's brain because it regulates DNA for genetic expression. *It is not genes or DNA that controls or regulates your biology, but the environment that regulates your genes.* This new revolutionary idea is called "epigenetics" (or, non-genetic factors that cause an organism's genes to behave or "express themselves" differently). It is time to stop blaming your genes on your ancestors. You have a lot of control over your genetic expression through your diet, thoughts, belief system, and the choice of actions you take.

Mankind's Attempts to "Measure"

NASA's Wilkinson Microwave Anisotropy Probe (WMAP) Spacecraft expedition in 2003 revealed vital information about our universe. The age of the universe is estimated at 13.7 billion years made up of:

- 4 percent matter (stars, planets, and gas, etc.)
- 23 percent exotic "dark matter" (detectable by its gravity)
- 73 percent "dark energy" (detectable by antigravity force)

The size of the universe is unknown. It is expanding and really big. The shape of the universe is perfectly flat—like a pizza.

With the best detectable scientific instrument, we can only measure 4 percent of matter in the universe. Ninety-six percent of the universe is considered to be made of "dark matter and dark energy," which means we don't know what it is, but it is out there. With the best medical scientific instrument, we can only measure a small fraction of the human being in a form of an x-ray, a CT scan, an MRI, a PET scan, or several other imaging devices created to "monitor" or "map."

New medicine based on new understanding of biology is here to challenge the basis of Western medicine, which has been dominated by a Newtonian mechanistic view of the causes and effects of health and illness (See: What is a Newtonian Mechanistic View of Causes and Effects?"). Modern biomechanical- and biochemical-based medical science cannot adequately describe the body, mind, and spirit of mankind. We have successfully dissected and studied until we have compartmentalized specialties of medicine, psychiatry, and religion, but we have never really studied a "whole living person" (or a unique individual called a man—or a woman). Given that we have never studied a whole person, what happens when we develop illness or chronic dis-ease?

Is There Such a Thing as a Chronic or Incurable Disease?

Why is it so difficult to treat chronic disease? Is there such a thing as an "incurable disease?" An incurable disease can be defined as a condition that is not curable by traditional Western medicine or alternative medical care—for that particular medical problem. In my practice, I have helped many patients suffering from conditions considered incurable by utilizing Acupuncture Meridian Assessment to uncover the disturbance of their biocybernetic matrix and by correcting their biological terrain. A person's "terrain" is the soil, or the internal bodily

---

What Is a Newtonian Mechanistic View of Causes and Effects?

Isaac Newton (1643-1727) and René Descartes (1596–1650) are credited for laying the groundwork for a belief known as "mechanistic philosophy." From the 17th century on, the dominant worldview has been that nature can be explained in the same way we understand the workings of a machine. Mechanism sees the universe as one great system made of separate interlocking parts.

This view sees the parts of the machine working together and obeying a few simple laws that can be predicted and measured. Unfortunately, for humans, the mechanistic view holds that the workings of the universe are no longer governed by God or for human purposes, but rather are determined by a mechanical interaction of inanimate objects obeying universal mathematical laws of cause and effect.

By the end of the 20th century, the mechanistic view was well established in what we now call classical physics. Due to its adoption in mainstream scientific circles, mechanism spread rapidly to the life sciences. Mechanism discourages all scientific inquiry, other than that which is linear, and is incremental as well as amenable to observation, calculation, and prediction.

Note: With its emphasis on "predictable data," evidence-based medicine, described in the previous chapter, is an example of mechanism.

environment that maintains them and keeps them strong. Correcting a terrain often involves:

- Changing diet

- Taking supplements with targeted nutrition

- Eliminating allergies and environmental toxicity

- Identifying dental problems

- Eradicating parasites

Many of the case studies described in this book are examples of patients whose health problems disappeared when their bodies' terrain was corrected.

Incurable patients have complex medical problems, and some have underlying and unresolved emotional conflicts. Among these patients, it could be said that their incurable condition is not necessarily a true medical problem. If this is the case, their expectations will never be fulfilled, and they will never be satisfied. Their journey of looking for a solution involves doctor visit after doctor visit—and, quite often, they expect to be disappointed. These people may even need failure at the subconscious level. An incurable patient is not the same as an incurable disease. Is there hope for incurable patients?

Many "incurable patients" need an honest self-evaluation, as well as counseling, to assess their inner conflict with their body, mind, and spirit. Their incurable medical conditions may have originated as unresolved emotional states from childhood, or possibly dead-end marriages or careers. This does not mean "it is all in their heads." However, patients' emotional states affect their health, and unresolved conflicts are embedded in every cell of their bodies (100 trillion cells), resonating and manifesting in their organs.

The Emotional Side of an Illness

For most physicians, dealing with a patient's fear and managing stress is the most challenging part of a medical practice. It is not so much how much stress you have, but rather how you deal with the stress. Anger and resentment may manifest in liver and gallbladder dysfunction. Emotional shock may trigger a heart attack. Fear and grief may suppress the immune system. Anxiety and loneliness may affect digestive function. In this sense, we do not age in a linear time scale by months and years, but by events and our emotional reaction to them.

If an incurable patient's emotional conflict can be beneficially resolved, they may experience "spontaneous" healing when all medical therapies have failed. The removal of suppressed guilt, fear, anger, shame, or self-doubt can trigger a major shift in one's hormonal, psychological, and immune response. Conventional medical professionals often dismiss this phenomenon as a placebo effect or, at best, a spontaneous healing. In spite of this view, there is ample evidence that the resolution of a strong emotional conflict can allow the body to heal itself.

I hope you had a chance to read the entire book so you have a better understanding of the concepts of biological terrain, biocybernetics, and how Acupuncture Meridian Assessment (AMA) and quantum physics are related to the biology of man. Many short essays, case studies, and testimonials, which I have added to this book, will give you tips on how to help yourself and your family. I sincerely hope that this book will guide you through your journey of healing. As I mentioned previously in this chapter, each person's healing process has its own unique time scale.

One of my favorite essays is "80% Solution for 20% of the Problem: What a Crock Pot Idea!" that metaphorically compares the human body to a violin that is part of a symphony called *life*. The same essay compares human experience to cooking in a crock pot (a rather wacky idea). The water in the pot is like emotion that holds the essence of life. How we stir the water in the pot gives us the final flavor of what it means to have a unique human experience.

What Is a Placebo Effect?

Placebos are sugar pills or saline injections that are given to patients in place of drugs that result in therapeutic improvement. The improvement is thought to be due to a patient's faith in their doctor.

Patients Ask About My Success Rate

Patients always ask me questions such as "Have you seen a case like mine? What is your success rate?" My usual answer is "You are *it*! There is no one like you in this planet with 6 billion people, and there are no statistics to guide or misguide you." You create your own variables for success or failure. When patients ask whether I can help them, my typical answer is "Maybe yes, maybe no." As a physician, I educate, coach, and train my patients how to prioritize and eliminate their problems in the right sequence, and I get them to think about the fact that healing must come from within. Healing is dependent on a person's belief system, attitude, and positive actions that lead to what medicine calls "spontaneous healing." The spontaneous healing that I'm describing is *not* what the medical establishment likes to call a placebo effect (See: "What Is a Placebo Effect?"). Rather, healing is based on new medicine based on new biology.

In the quantum world, everything is uncertain and everything can influence everything else and everything is possible. When you come to see me for an evaluation, be prepared for the quantum world of uncertainty. I will check your biocybernetic matrix system comprising acupuncture meridians. Your medical problems may not be what you think, what you have been told, or what has been diagnosed. My recommendation might be unusual or weird at first, but most likely it will make more sense to you later. I am not responsible for your cure. Let's call it *accidental cure*. Why not!

Notes

About the Author

Dr. Simon Yu, M.D

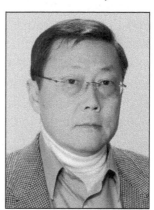

Dr. Simon Yu practices internal medicine and alternative complementary medicine in St. Louis, Missouri. After completing an undergraduate degree from Washington University, Dr. Yu earned a master's degree on influenza virus and cell-mediated immunology from the University of Missouri at St. Louis in research work he completed at Washington University. He later graduated from the University of Missouri at Columbia School of Medicine in 1984 and completed an internal medicine residency at St. Mary's Health Center in St. Louis. In 2006, Dr. Yu retired as a full colonel from the Army Reserve. The extra time afforded him an ability to take 300 hours of acupuncture training from Stanford University's School of Medicine.

Background in Alternative/Complementary Medicine

Dr. Yu worked as a regional medical director at a large HMO medical group for 10 years and has been studying alternative/complementary medicine for the last 20 years.

Career Milestone: Dr. Cook's Energy Medicine Conference, 1996

In the Foreword to Dr. Douglas Cook's new book, *Rescued By My Dentist*, Dr. Yu provides details about a 1996 dental and medical conference that totally transformed his career. Dr. Douglas Cook, who practices dentistry in a Wisconsin town that had a population of 605 in the 2000 census, was sponsoring one of his many Chicago-based conferences that he titled "Conference on Energy in Medicine and Dentistry." Dr. Yu was one of a small number of medical doctors who attended the conference. He quotes Dr. Tom Stone, another M.D. at the conference, who succinctly stated what Dr. Yu felt was his own reason for attending the conference:

To find out how dentists are killing my patients.

Until Dr. Yu attended Dr. Cook's conference, he did not realize the magnitude of the relationship between the oral cavity's pathology and patient health.

At the 1996 conference, Dr. Cook introduced his conference participants to computerized electrodermal screening (CEDS) that Dr. Yu later renamed Acupuncture Meridian Assessment (and describes several times in this book).

Dr. Yu says he was skeptical at first and took a second CEDS conference before realizing that Rhinehold Voll's tool (an EAV device) provides a medical doctor or dentist a valuable method for evaluating the connections between the teeth and the body. Once he began to use an EAV device in his practice, Dr. Yu understood that energy meridians and energy fields can totally transform a medical practice. As he says, "Medicine became fun." Ironically, he had to study dentistry to learn about medical illness.

For doctors or patients who would like to reach Dr. Cook:

Douglas Cook, DDS
10971 Clinic Road
Suring, Wisconsin 54174
Phone: (920) 842-2083
www.dentistryhealth.com

Career Milestone: U.S. Army Reserve Mission, Bolivia, 2001

Dr. Cook's CEDS conferences placed Dr. Yu in a small group of American physicians who understand the connection between oral pathology and illness. A few years later, his career as an Army Reservist took him on a mission to Bolivia where he made a discovery that placed him in an *even smaller* group of physicians who understand the connection between *parasites and disease.*

As described in Chapter 6, most American medical doctors hardly have any experience with parasites or experience using parasite medications. Bolivia provided a rapid education over a 2-week period in several small towns where the U.S. government dispensed antiparasite medications to approximately 10,000 Andes Indians. As Dr. Yu states in Chapter 6:

> *The key part of my story occurred within days after the first group of Indians was treated with antiparasite medications. Several patients returned to relay stories of seeing parasites passing in their stools and a few had parasites erupt from their skin. Their stories, the samples they brought in jars, and their descriptions of how much better they were feeling left me with what later turned out to be an important question: How much chronic illness is due to parasite infection?*

After returning to St. Louis, Dr. Yu learned to search for parasites with an EAV device. He also used parasite medications in various combinations and observed dramatic responses in patients whose illnesses were considered incurable. Some of the difficult conditions that responded with parasite medications include: intractable allergies and asthma, migraine headache, sciatica, constipation and diarrhea, irritable bowel syndrome, colitis, bronchiectasis, vision loss, anxiety, depression, nightmares, temporomandibular joint (TMJ) problems, chronic fatigue, fibromyalgia, multiple sclerosis, arthralgia and myalgia, pelvic pain, eczema, psoriasis, hypertension, and cancers.

Biological Dentists, St. Louis, Missouri

The following biological dentists (in alphabetical order) understand the connection between oral pathology and disease:

Stewart E. Moreland, D.M.D., for oral surgery
2821 N. Ballas Road, Suite 225
St. Louis, Missouri 63131
(314) 569-1012
www.drsmoreland.com
info@drsmoreland.com

Michael G. Rehme, D.D.S., C.C.N.
2821 North Ballas Rd, Suite 245
St. Louis, Missouri 63131
(314) 997-2550
www.toothandbodyconnection.com

Ron Schoolman, D.D.S.
16976 Old Manchester Rd
Wildwood, Missouri 63040
(314) 458-9090
cherryhillsdental.com
info@cherryhillsdental.com

Gary B. Wiele, D.D.S.
950 Francis Place, Suite 311
Clayton, Missouri 63105
(314) 726-2265
www.stlouisdentist.biz

Index

4-dimethylaminoazobenzene (DAB), butter yellow, 162, 163

A

Abraham, Dr. Guy E., Optimox Corporation, author, medical journal and Web articles (search Amazon.com), 204
Accelerated aging, 222, 240, 267
Achoff, Dr. Dieter, 389
Acid reflux, 186, 263, 273, 325
Acne, 143, 238, 267, 338, 369
Acupuncture Meridian Assessment (AMA), 26-29, 32-33, 49, 53, 55, 59-60, 62, 64, 90, 110-111, 113-114, 116, 118, 224, 283, 285, 299, 304-305, 342, 351, 368, 283, 393-394, 396, 410-411, 417, 420, 452
Acupuncture, 27, 31, 48-49, 53-56, 58, 60, 93, 228, 265, 275, 285, 300, 304, 395, 421
ADD/ADHD, 59, 73, 143, 340-341
Adderall, 335, 339
ADHD drugs, CBS news story, 25% of college students taking ADHD drugs to focus, 340
Agatston, Dr. Arthur, author, book, *The South Beach Diet: the Delicious, Doctor Designed, Fool Proof Plan for Fast and Healthy Weight Loss,* 262
Agent Orange, 172
Allergies 26, 32-33, 44, 49, 74, 81, 90, 92, 110-111, 117-118, 140, 142-144, 174-175, 194-195, 198, 208, 224-226, 260, 262, 264, 268, 276, 284, 305-306, 311, 314, 317-319, 322-323, 327, 329, 340-341, 350, 352, 369-370, 373, 376, 388, 401, 410, 418
Allopathic medicine, 90, 124, 272, 275, 381, 386, 403
Alternative therapies, 33, 181, 244, 265, 275-276, 303, 450
Aluminum, 68, 73, 75, 77, 203, 293, 301, 310, 314, 327, 346
Alzheimer's disease, the most common form of dementia, thought to reach 107 million people by 2050, 68, 77, 275, 324, 372
Amalgams, 43, 67-70, 79, 82-83, 101, 208-209, 268, 286-287, 293-294, 306, 309-310, 312-313, 339, 342-346, 350, 401
Amati, Nicolo, an Italian luthier (violin maker) from Cremona whose violins are considered suitable for modern playing, 55
American Association of Endodontists, 87, 101, 362
American Cancer Society, 272, 380
American Cancer Society, reported rate of cancer deaths, 272
American College of Advancement in Medicine (ACAM), 69
American Dental Association (ADA), 82-83, 343
American Diabetes Association, 150

* Author has written several books

* Author has written several books

* Author has written several books

C

* Author has written several books

* Author has written several books

* Author has written several books

E

* Author has written several books

F

* Author has written several books

G

* Author has written several books

* Author has written several books

H

* Author has written several books

* Author has written several books

* author has written several books

* Author has written several books

* Author has written several books

M

* Author has written several books

N

* Author has written several books

* Author has written several books

* Author has written several books

* Author has written several books

S

* Author has written several books

* Author has written several books

T

* Author has written several books

* Author has written several books

W

* Author has written several books

X

Y

Z

* Author has written several books

Recommended Reading

Articles, *The Healthy Planet*

The Healthy Planet magazine, now in its thirteenth year, was founded by J.B. Lester and his wife, Niki. This section is a guide to Dr. Yu's *Healthy Planet* articles that have not been included in his book but are beneficial to read. Look for the following titles, which are archived on his Web site (www.preventionandhealing.com).

Obtaining Acrobat Reader

The articles on Dr. Yu's Web site open in Adobe Acrobat Reader. If you do not have the Adobe Acrobat Reader software, you can get it for free by clicking on the "Get Acrobat Reader" icon. This will take you to Adobe's website and enable you to download the free Acrobat Reader program to your computer. If you are not sure if you have this software, try clicking on one of the articles. You'll quickly find out if it opens in this software.

- "Accidental Cure, the Book, Challenging Medical Informatics and Evidence Based Medicine"
- "Acupuncture and Acupuncture Meridian Assessment: Journey to East by West"
- "Awakening the Healer Within You: Medical Spiritual Wellness from a Bucket of KFC"
- "Basal Temperature Test—Check Thyroid Activity"
- "Biological Terrain"
- "Biological Terrain Revisited: Balancing Acid/Base, Oxidation Potential, and More"
- "(Adrenal) Burnout Syndrome—Last Stage of Exhaustion"
- "Color Me Blue Color Me Red: Biocybernetics and Color Medicine Conference in St. Louis"
- "Combat Medical Care and Holistic Medicine"

- "Congestive Heart Failure: Nutrition, Infection, Drugs, and Environmental Failure"
- "Crohns Disease and Ulcerative Colitis: Think Parasite, Allergies and More Parasites?"
  (Note: See the related patient success Story—"Success Story: Crohn's Disease—How do you thank a man who has saved the life of your child?")
- "Cure for All Diseases and Non-Diseases: Let's Start with Honey Bee Erectile Dysfunction"
- "Death by (Modern) Medicine: White Coats as a Symbol of Life and Death"
- "Diabetes Epidemic—Evolutionary Adaptation to Food Crime"
- "Disappearance of the Universe as We Know It for WIMPs: What If a Cancer Patient Doesn't Really Have Cancer?"
- "Duh Vinci Code for Tasmanian Devils: Cracking the Cancer Code"
- "Each New Season Calls for Cleansing and Detoxification
- "Gateway to German Biological Medicine: Saint Louis to Baden Baden, Germany via Canada"
- "German Biological Medicine: Leading the World in Natural Healing"
- "Healing Crisis by Herxheimer Reaction: Is This Side Effects or Lazarus Effects?"
- "Healing Foods from the Bible: Jesus Did Not Eat Junk Food"
- "Heart Rate Variability—New Way to Evaluate Physical Fitness"
- "Heidelberg pH Gastric Acid Analysis: For Acid Reflux, Allergies, Belching, IBS, Or Gas Problems"
- "Holistic Exercise Program and the 'Five Rites'"
- "House of Wonder by a Quack: Upton Sinclair on Abrams and Frequency Specific Micro-Current"
- "Hypertension: How to Silence the Great Killer"
- "Hypoglycemia—the Great Masquerader"
- "Hypothyroidism—Unsuspected Cause for Fatigue and Obesity"

- "Luthiers and Physicians: Living Life by a Symphony of Strings and Meridians"
- "Lyme Disease, Autism and Beyond: Is This Just Another New Fad or a New Modern Plague?"
- "Maximus and Minimus: Cure for All, Cure for None"
- "Medical Infrared Thermography: Heat Recognition from Tanks to Tumors"
- "Migraine Headache Puzzle: Migration of Headache Along the Meridians"
- Molds—Enigma of Indoor Pollution
- "New Medicine Based on New Biology: Maybe Yes, Maybe No One Hundred Dollar Cure: Cure for Braves, Skeptics and El Cheapo"
- "The Original Incurable: The Gifted Village Idiot in the Holistic Medical Community"
- "Parasites and Allergies—Paradise Lost in a Parallel Universe"
- "Parasites and Mental Illness"
- "Parasites and Mind Control"
- "Parasites Down Under from This Wormy World: De-worming from Silk Road to Boeing 747 and Airbus 380"
- "Parasites, Inflammation and Cancer: Ring of Fire Feeding Tumor Cells"
- "Parasites Speak Many Languages"
- "Raw Food Smoothie Immune Rejuvenation Diet—Based on Teachings of Dr. Wu, Yu"
- "RNA Based Nutrigenomic Therapy: New Treatment for Autism and Neuro-Degenerative Disease"
- "Ten Dollar Cure When One Hundred Dollar Cure Fails: Wheat Belly, Corn Butt and More or Less"
- "Ten Golden Rules for Wellness"
- "The Truth About Anti-aging and Hormone Replacement Therapy"
- "Think Dental When the Latest Medical Therapy Fails: Mouth Battery, High Speed Drill, and Others"

- "Water, Salt and Human Energy"
- "Who Is Afraid of Hulda Clark?"
- "Wisdom Teeth, Undetected Tooth Infections and Incurable Medical Symptoms"

In-Depth Articles

All of the following articles are written by Dr. Yu. They are intended to educate new and current patients on the Alternative and Complementary medicine viewpoint of the symptoms or illness described.

- "ADD / ADHD"
- "Attention Deficit Disorder / Attention Deficit Hyperactivity Disorder"
- "Arthritis and Chronic Pain"
- "Reversing Degenerative Arthritis with Nutritional Therapy"
- "Cancer—Nutritional Therapies for Cancer"
- "Chronic Fatigue"
- "Fibromyalgia (Myofascial Pain Syndrome)"
- "Optimal Health Maintenance Recommendations"
- "Osteoporosis—Preventing and Reversing Osteoporosis"
- "Peak Performance Diet"
- "Yeast Syndrome"

Books

In the last twenty years, mergers and acquisitions in the book publishing industry have caused large book publishers to scale very large. Most of today's large book publishers are owned by media companies interested in books related to the movie industry—making it very difficult for alternative medical doctors to find publishers. The same media companies that own large publishing firms also rent space in large retail bookstores. Although large retailers have devoted shelf space to alternative healing, the health section of most book stores is dominated by authors who write conventional books. Many alternative health practitioners have relied on health food stores to sell their books when other avenues of distribution were closed.

To assist readers, young doctors, teachers, students, librarians, and the general reading public learn the titles of books written by devoted alternative health practitioners, I have created this recommended book section with books arranged alphabetically by title. Each page contains reasons why I think you should buy these books.

—Simon Yu, M.D.

In 1994, Amy Lansky was a senior computer scientist working at NASA when her son Max became one among a growing number of autistic children around the world. In her quest to find a cure for her son, Lansky discovered an amazing medical treatment from America's past that is now the second-most-used medical modality in the world—*homeopathy*. Within days of beginning treatment in early 1995, Max began showing subtle but noticeable signs of improvement. Over the next two years, he gradually reached nearly complete recovery, and by the time he was ten years old,

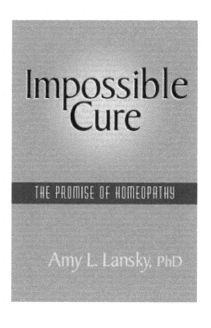

Max was cured. This remarkable experience led Dr. Lansky to study homeopathy and become one of its leading advocates in the US. She also wrote a book to enable others to learn about the miraculous healing power of this amazing form of medical treatment.

Impossible Cure: The Promise of Homeopathy is a general introduction to homeopathy that provides an in-depth and exciting account of the history, philosophy, science, and experience of homeopathic medicine. Since it appeared in 2003, it has consistently been one of the best-selling books on homeopathy around the world. It is used not only as a patient education book but also as an introductory textbook at several homeopathic schools. It has also been translated into German, Greek, Arabic, and Czech.

One of the key features of *Impossible Cure* is its use of illustrative first-person testimonials. The most significant is the amazing story of how Amy Lansky's son was cured of autism. But the book also includes dozens of other testimonials of homeopathic cures for a variety of physical, mental, and emotional conditions.

Impossible Cure will serve as an invaluable guide to anyone interested in learning more about this intriguing form of health care. To learn more about Impossible Cure and about homeopathic treatment (especially the treatment of autism), please visit www.impossiblecure.com.

An introduction to homeopathy that stands out from the rest.

—Dr. Joseph Mercola
Mercola Newsletter

The finest general introduction to homeopathy I've yet read... This book should be read by everyone interested in homeopathy, from the rank beginner to the seasoned professional. It has something new in it for everyone.

—Julian Winston
Editor, *Homeopathy Today*;
Author, *The Faces of Homeopathy*

We have never had this kind of response to an introductory book.

—Greg Cooper
Owner, Minimum Price
Homeopathic Books

An accessible guide to one of the most mysterious of healing arts.

—Wayne B. Jonas, MD
Director, Samueli Institute;
Former director, Office of Alternative
Medicine, NIH

This book may very well contribute to the transformation of homeopathy from the ugly duckling of medicine to the swan that it deserves to be.

—Lia Bello, RN, FNP, CCH,
Reviewer for *Homeopathy Today*

D r. David Brownstein, author of *Iodine: Why You Need It, Why You Can't Live Without It*, is an extraordinary physician-researcher who has pieced together a connection that exists between endocrine-related illnesses and iodine supplies in the body (illnesses that include cancer). Remarkably, nineteenth century physicians knew of the importance of iodine and frequently prescribed a solution of iodine, potassium iodide, and water developed in 1829 by a French physician named Jean Lugol, who named the liquid Lugol's solution.

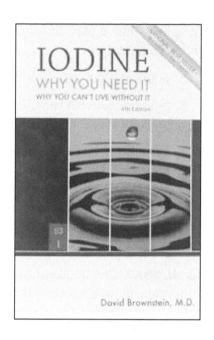

Brownstein and a handful of other doctors, who are leading what is known as The Iodine Project, are sounding an important alarm that warns us that we need more iodine. Early twentieth century public health officials discovered a clue about iodine deficiency in the nation's goiter belts, but the iodized salt that was introduced as a solution for this deficiency supplies an insufficient amount of iodine for what is a long list of non-thyroid functions.

Most of today's medical practitioners are clueless about the body's many needs for iodine and that the reduced forms of other halides (bromine, chlorine, and fluorine) can block iodine uptake in the body. Although many people have heard of fluoride, chloride, and possibly even bromide, the health problems caused by these toxic minerals, located in a column of the periodic table known as the halogen family, are almost universally ignored. Brownstein writes:

> *Bromine intoxication has been shown to cause delirium, psychomotor retardation, schizophrenia and hallucination. Subjects who ingest enough bromine feel dull and apathetic and have difficulty concentrating.*

In spite of this effect, bromine (or its reduced form—bromide) is used indiscriminately in:

- pools and hot tubs as a disinfectant

- pharmaceuticals (inhalers, nasal sprays, a nerve gas antidote, and a bladder medication)

- agriculture as fumigant for termites and other pests

- bread as a dough conditioner

- soft drinks as an emulsifier to help natural fat-soluble citrus flavors stay suspended in the drink (e.g., Mountain Dew, AMP Energy Drink, and some Gatorade drinks)

Dr. Brownstein's outstanding book explains that iodine's non-thyroid functions include a role in the detoxification of heavy metals and toxic halides as well as a natural elimination of malfunctioning cells (called apoptosis or programmed cell death). We need authors like Dr. Brownstein to point out toxic minerals that slip through government scrutiny, as well as Nature's solutions!

D r. Hal A. Huggins' book *It's All in Your Head: The Link Between Mercury Amalgams and Illness* is worth its weight in gold. The book contains paradigm-shifting information and step-by-step solutions for mercury toxicity from dental amalgams that have been thwarted by special interests for many years. The key to this crime appears on the book's last page:

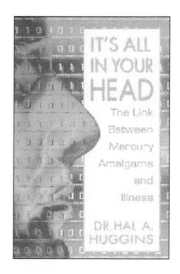

As of this writing (1993), in all states except California, dentists are threatened with the loss of their license to practice if they so much as mention to a patient that mercury might be hazardous.

The expression "hindsight is better than foresight" is a proverb that is supposed to express a simple truth, but what if hindsight is deliberately blocked by controlling interests for over 170 years? Dr. Huggins was first introduced to the dangers of mercury by Dr. Olympio Pinto of Rio de Janiero in 1973 and soon learned that mercury had been debated in dental circles since the 1830s with a voracity that he characterized as Amalgam Wars One, Two, and Three.

In the nineteenth century, the National Association of Dental Surgeons became a casualty of Amalgam War One when they banned, as unethical, any dentist who used mercury. Amalgam War Two was led by a German chemist named Dr. Alfred Stock who published over thirty articles condemning the use of amalgam. Although Stock's research gained recognition in Europe, he was discredited by the dental community and lost his records in a bombing during World War II. Dr. Huggins says he started Amalgam War Three after Dr. Pinto briefed him about his own research. Pinto had compiled the largest bibliography on mercury toxic-ity while working on a master's degree at Georgetown University, but the National Institute of Dental Research (NIDR) forced Georgetown to have Pinto stopped. Huggins' stories about what followed are so horrific it's amazing that he had the stamina to persevere. Dr. Robert Atkins, who wrote the book's foreword, calls Huggins a "pioneer courageous enough to charge full tilt at the fortified ramparts of conventional medical care."

In spite of a very difficult path, Huggins' accomplishments and research are beautifully chronicled in this amazing book. Milestones include:

- Measurement of electrical current in the mouth and the health-threatening consequences of negative current
- Discovery of toxic vapor emitted from mercury amalgams with a Bacharach mercury detector borrowed from the Department of Health
- Use of immunological reactivity testing to mercury that Huggins first carried out for his master's degree that he completed at age fifty-two
- Identification of methyl mercury, a compound formed in the mouth that is one hundred times more toxic than elemental mercury
- Recognition that methylation, the chemical process in the mouth that produces methyl mercury, is accelerated in negative current
- Acknowledgment that Dr. Olympio Pinto (Mexico City, 1973) is correct about mercury's threat to sulfhydryl groups in the body's proteins, including blood serum proteins
- Establishment of a laboratory where physicians and dentists all over the world can have dental materials tested
- Classification of medical diseases that occur as a result of dental amalgam that span five categories (neurological, cardiovascular, collagen, immunological, and miscellaneous)
- Success with incapacitating neurological diseases such as MS, ALS, Alzheimer's, and Lupus
- Discovery of positive ALS patient response when cavitations are opened and the periodontal ligament is removed
- Identification of measurable parameters in blood chemistry that constitute early warning signs of mercury toxicity
- Use of urine porphyrin testing as a test for toxicities from mercury, braces, root canals, chrome crowns, nickel crowns, and amalgams

- Realization that cholesterol is an important constituent in cell membranes and hormones, in addition to the fact that mercury can interfere with the production of succinic acid, a building block for cholesterol
- Creation of a total protein (albumin and globulin)-to-globulin ratio used to determine the speed of patient recovery (patients with a ratio below 2.6 respond slowly)
- Discovery that Vitamin A, minerals, and digestive enzymes are factors that speed recovery, with Vitamin A as a key factor
- Use of hair analysis as a diagnostic tool for mercury toxicity and deranged mineral disposition that results from exposure to toxic metals
- Identification of elevated blood enzymes alkaline phosphatase (alk phos) and lactic dehydrogenase (LDH) as indicators of mercury toxicity
- Clinical observation that patients with severe MS, epilepsy, or emotional disease usually have six or more negative-current fillings
- Use of sequential amalgam removal as an effective way to remove mercury fillings within a quadrant with the highest negative fillings removed first
- Use of absolute sequential amalgam removal in patients with leukemia or ALS—in descending order from high negative to low positive
- Identification of a 7-14-21-day immune cycle as a predictor of low-immune defense days during patient recovery
- Discovery of low body temperature in patients whose thyroid hormone has mercury attached at iodine activation sites
- Recognition of black streaks in retinas of mercury toxic patients
- Dietary supplementation determination through blood test results
- Use of a bubble operatory design that reduces mercury vapor during active procedures from 880 micrograms per cubic meter to zero

In her best-selling cookbook *Nourishing Traditions*, nutrition journalist Sally Fallon Morell exposes current establishment low-fat propaganda as a conspiracy to rob Americans of their health and vitality, and to enrich the powerful food processing industry, based in large part on refined carbohydrates and vegetable oils derived from corn and soybeans.

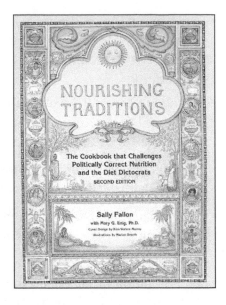

Sally and her colleague, Mary G. Enig, Ph.D., a world-renowned expert on the subject of lipids and human nutrition, draw on a wealth of scientific and anthropological findings to refute the notion that Americans should cut back on animal fats and cholesterol-rich foods, pointing out that animal fats and cholesterol are not villains but vital factors in the diet, necessary for normal growth, proper function of the brain and nervous system, protection from disease, and optimum energy levels. Animal fats and proteins are especially necessary for the proper development of babies and children.

Other themes in *Nourishing Traditions* include the importance of traditional broths as a source of minerals and as an aid to digestion, made from the bones of chicken, fish, beef, and lamb; of proper preparation of grains, nuts, and legumes to neutralize enzyme inhibitors and mineral-blocking substances found in all seed foods; and of ancient techniques for food preservation that enhance nutrient content while supplying beneficial digestive flora on a daily basis.

Fallon Morell explains the importance of returning to organic farming, pasture-fed livestock, and whole traditional foods, properly prepared, if Americans are to regain their health and vitality, as well as the benefits of an economy based on small-scale organic production and food processing that returns added value to the independent farmer, rather than to large-scale food processing conglomerates.

Dr. Douglas Cook, D.D.S., is, perhaps, the most distinguished author in this group of authors whose books I am reviewing, due to his *fifty-seven years* in dentistry and his contributions that are beautifully described in his book *Rescued by My Dentist: New Solutions to a Health Crisis.* Due to his length of service, he is fortunate to have known, and taken three seminars from, Dr. Reinhold Voll, M.D. (1908–1989), who developed Electro Acupuncture According to Voll (EAV), on which my work in now based. Besides writing a wonderful book,

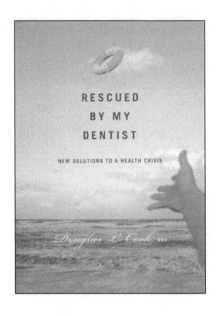

Dr. Cook has also presented over twenty seminars on dental material and EAV in Asia, Mexico, Australia, Canada, and the Untied States. I met Dr. Cook at one of those seminars in 1996, and, as I've described in my book, the experience changed my career in medicine (see "About the Author," page 423).

Propelled by an observation that "there is a need to help patients suffering from illnesses directly related to the oral cavity," Dr. Cook helped pioneer the use of an electro-medical procedure that helps dentists and doctors diagnose pathology in the mouth as well as the entire body. In Dr. Cook's book, EAV is called computerized electro-dermal screening (CEDS). Courses in CEDS (or EAV) are available from the American Association of Acupuncture and Bio-Energetic Medicine (AAABEM), which is headquartered in Honolulu, Hawaii (www.ibemedicine.com/lamclinicinc.html).

Mercury is a major topic in Dr. Cook's book as it is in mine. Like all dentists and doctors, Dr. Cook had to discover the details about mercury toxicity on his own. Remarkably, Dr. Cook read about mercury toxicity in an article titled "Quicksilver and Slow Death" by John J. Putman that was published in the October 1972 edition of *National Geographic* magazine![1]

Dr. Cook devotes sections to oral galvanism, high-speed drilling, root canals, and cavitations, presenting interesting stories about people and events that shaped his learning experiences. His book is a gem that is filled with generous insights from a veteran who has been searching for nearly six decades. Biological dentists and alternative medical doctors will understand the challenges Dr. Cook encountered in the search for new developments as well as the time required for self-study. For example, in chapter 1 and chapter 4, Dr. Cook relays startling information about the dangers of high-speed drilling that he learned in a week long seminar given by Drs. Ed Arana, D.D.S., Ralph Turk, and Fritz Kramer in September 1987. During the seminar, Dr. Turk presented slides showing dental nerve damage and bacterial infection that result from high-speed drills. Later that year (twenty-four years ago), Dr. Cook replaced his high-speed drill with a 20,000 revolution per minute drill that reduces sensitivity and helps save teeth. This safer, conservative approach is a sharp contrast to conventional high-speed drilling, which runs at 350,000 revolutions per minute. High-speed drills create vacuums that pull odontoblasts out of dentinal tubules, allowing bacteria to pass through the tubules, causing infection and death of the teeth.

Because alternative health practitioners have a frequent need to substantiate any developments that are contrary to the mainstream, Dr. Cook has provided an impressive array of scientific journal

---

1 In 2000, the U.S. Department of the Interior and the U.S. Geological Survey published "Mercury Recycling in the United States," which is available as a PDF file on the Web (http://pubs.usgs.gov/circ/c1196u/circ_1196_U.pdf). It cites John Putman's article in the references. Authors William E. Brooks and Grecia R. Matos refer to "Ever-increasing human health and envionemental concerns" and include the following recommendation: "continued substitution of nonmercury replacement devices and materials for automobile convenience switches, dental amalgams, fluorescent lamps, medical devices, thermometers, and thermostats may reduce the secondary supply of mercury for recycling." Note: The FDA and ADA are both silent on this issue.

references for each chapter of his book. *Rescued by My Dentist: New Solutions to a Health Crisis* is available in print on Amazon.com and as an e-book on Dr. Cook's Web site at www.dentistryhealth.com.

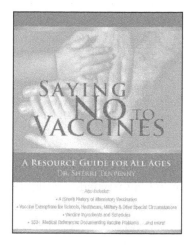

D r. Sherri Tenpenny's *Saying No to Vaccines: A Resource Guide for All Ages* is a book that has the power to save lives. For many, this statement will cause what psychologists call cognitive dissonance. Dissonance refers to a clash, and cognitive dissonance refers to tension that results when new information conflicts with a previously existing belief. Dr. Russell Blaylock, M.D., who wrote the foreword to the book, warns readers that when they "enter this controversial area (vaccines), naive worldviews go out the window."

For example, readers may be startled to learn that in the nineteenth century, some of the most severe epidemics in Europe occurred after an onset of compulsory vaccinations. Sherri questions the science of vaccinations and quotes researcher D.L. Perry, who wrote for an early edition of the *British Medical Journal*:

> *How is it that smallpox is five times as likely to be fatal in the vaccinated as in the unvaccinated?*

Today, there are so many vaccine mandates and so much coercion applied that who, but a few courageous authors, would dare to draw attention to the fact that there are epidemics among the vaccinated? Or that vaccines cause fatalities? Sherri has become so thoroughly versed on this topic that she has appeared as an expert witness in the U.S. Federal Court of Claims, nicknamed the "Vaccine Court," where more than $1 billion has been paid to vaccine-injured victims. In chapter 3, where Sherri refutes the twenty-five most common arguments supporting vaccines, she explains that vaccine failure rates are between 24 and 38 percent, and that outbreaks have occurred in populations where vaccination coverage approached 100%.

The key to why the vaccinations have not been discontinued in spite of severe adverse reactions is described in the same chapter:

The global vaccine business is projected to grow 18% per year, well above the 4.4% annual growth expected from the drug industry overall (vaccines are manufactured by pharmaceutical companies).

One of the most serious warnings in Sherri's book is that dozens of vaccines are in the manufacturing pipeline and destined to become *mandates* for children, adolescents, and adults in the next few years. She explains that there has been a struggle between the pro-vaccination and anti-vaccination forces since the first compulsory vaccines (150 years ago), but the situation has changed. Today, the clout of the pharmaceutical giants is used to persuade and coerce state and national government officials to embrace massive, expensive vaccination programs.

Sherri's contribution is enormous, and she does not just point at a problem. In chapter 4, she presents detailed information about four types of exemptions that may be used to legally avoid vaccinations (philosophical, religious, medical, and proof of immunity). Surprisingly, many school administrators and pediatricians are not even aware that exemptions exist because so few parents request them. This chapter will help readers understand how these examptions compare, including possible landmines surrounding each of the exemptions. For example, although medical exemptions are allowed in fifty states, this would require a letter from an M.D. or D.O. who, as Dr. Blaylock says, is "willing to stand up to the vaccine juggernaut." Most states accept medical-exemption letters without question, but some letters are reviewed by a state employee with power to revoke an exemption. The other types of exemptions are accepted in some states, but not in others. Sherri has done an excellent job of helping readers to understand the potential traps. Because vaccines are becoming a condition for college entrance and for employment, this chapter is valuable to both parents and a growing number of adults.

Sherri's book also includes twenty-four addendums that contain a volume of hard-to-obtain information. Due to her training as an osteopathic physician, Sherri has also included tips for minimizing the risk, including details for scheduling vaccines as well as a very important pre-vaccination pre-treatment with Vitamin C and Vitamin A.

Vaccinations laws have changed, and they will continue to change. Sherri explains that more than two hundred vaccination laws, appropriation bills, and policies are considered during each state legislative session across the nation. As she points out in the beginning of her book:

> *Protecting the right to refuse vaccnation will require political vigilance and active participation on the part of all who want their right to choose.*

Thank you, Sherri, for educating us about this very important subject.

Jeffrey Smith's *Seeds of Deception* is a precious book that makes readers aware of reckless decisions being made in the biotech industry affecting the foods that we eat.

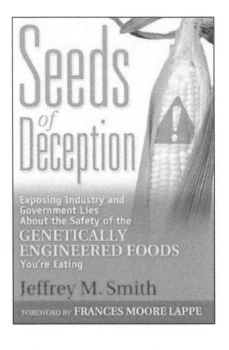

Jeffrey's thorough research uncovers the dark politics behind little-known missteps in genetic engineering that are underreported by the media.

This book is also an important reference guide to genetic engineering whistle-blowers and their stories. Examples include Árpád Pusztai, a Hungarian biochemist and nutritionist who was suspended from the Rowett Research Institute in Aberdeen, Scotland, when he told the truth about the effect genetically modified potatoes had on rats; Dr. Richard Burroughs, a veterinarian and senior FDA scientist who oversaw recombinant (genetically engineered) bovine growth hormone (rBGH) safety studies and was fired because his concerns about the safety of rBGH delayed the approval process of this hormone; Dr. Samuel Epstein, a British medical doctor and professor emeritus in environmental and occupational health at the University of Illinois at Chicago School of Public Health who has been targeted by a Monsanto-created hit squad, called the Dairy Coalition, that has pressured editors at the *Los Angeles Times*, the *Boston Globe*, the *Washington Post*, the *New York Times,* and the *Wall Street Journal*, warning them not to accept Epstein's articles about rGBH or any articles that cite his research; coauthors Marc Lappé and

Brit Bailey of the Center for Ethics and Toxics (CETOS); whose book, *Against the Grain, Biotechnology and the Corporate Takeover of Your Food*, was cancelled when Monsanto sent a threatening letter to their publisher; as well as Fox television reporters Jane Akre and her husband, Steve Wilson, who lost their jobs at WTVT in Tampa, Florida, when Monsanto pressured the station concerning their investigation about the dangers of rGBH.

Jeffrey's book needs to be promoted and endorsed by anyone who is concerned about the potential dangers of genetic engineering. His "What Could Go Wrong?" list in chapter 2 provides a helpful explanation of how scientists create synthetic genes and transfer them across natural species barriers. (Note: Since Jeffrey's book was published, a team, led by a scientist named Craig Venter, produced synthetic DNA and an entire cell on a computer in La Jolla, California in May 2010.)

Lax government regulations in the United States and the links between universities and industry are both important topics that are covered in Jeffrey's book. He quotes a *New Scientist* columnist who wrote:

> *Industry-based scientists have influence in high*
> *places—they move in the corridors of government.*

Be sure to memorize the year that the USDA tried to allow GMO ingredients into the definition of organic (1997). Jeffrey includes this embarrassing government proposal in a section titled "Does Organic Mean Non-GMO?" Animal lovers will be interested in the boxes at the end of each chapter containing stories about cows, hogs, squirrels, rats, elk, deer, raccoons, and mice who reject GMO food.

W hat could be better than reading a health book written by a natural medicine doctor who began his career in the 1970s? Dr. Jonathan Wright wrote the first prescription for bio-identical estrogen in the early 1980s, and his clinical experience with this antiaging therapy has been shared twice—first in 1997 with his *Natural Hormone Replacement for Women Over 45,* and again in 2010 with his *Stay Young and Sexy with Bio-Identical Hormone Replacement,* now in its second edition.

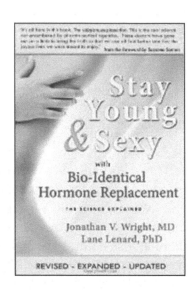

Dr. Wright and Dr. Lane Lenard, Ph.D., are prolific writers, and their contribution to natural medicine cannot be overstated.

Suzanne Somers, whose own books and star status helped draw attention to the benefits of bio-identical hormones on Oprah's and Dr. Phil's television shows in 2009, wrote this book's foreword, calling bio-identical hormone replacement "the backbone of anti-aging medicine."

One of the most fascinating stories in the book appears in a preface written by Dr. Wright titled, "Lessons from Ancient China." Amazingly, the ancient Chinese accomplished bio-identical hormone replacement between 1025 and 1833 AD. Wright calls this practice, the "first and finest job of copying nature" with bio-identical hormone replacement therapy (BHRT) and provides an intriguing overview of a very long list of hormones the Chinese administered in a precipitate made from the urine of young men and women that was compounded into pills. The hormone concentrate, produced by Taoist physicians, contained bio-identical estradiol, estriol, estrone, progesterone, DHEA, testostereone, and thyroid hormones that modern laboratories produce from plant precursors. The Chinese concentrate also contained a full complement of other human hormones that Wright acknowledges may not have yet been identified. Dr. Wright explains that the only part of modern BHRT that is superior to the early precipitate are transmucosal cremes that bypass the liver and carry hormones directly into the bloodstream.

The history of modern synthetic hormones is presented in their new book, as it was in the 1997 book, with additional comments on the unscheduled termination of the government's 2002 Women's Health Initiative (WHI) study that discredited patentable synthetic hormones. This event created a stampede away from synthetic hormones. Unfortunately, the WHI event also caused Wyeth Pharmaceuticals, has sold billions of dollars worth of synthetic hormones since the 1960s, to launch an unprecedented legal, lobbying, and public relations campaign to influence the FDA to eliminate hormones that are identical to nature.

By presenting the truth about synthetic hormones, this book provides a helpful glimpse into the politics of natural medicine as much as it explains the science behind bio-identical hormone therapy. In the book's last chapter, titled "The Politics of Bio-Identical Hormones," Wright and Lane present details of the FDA's ban of estriol, the natural estrogen that has an anticarcinogenic effect, as well as FDA harassment of compounding pharmacies that supply the public with bio-identical hormones.

Dr. Wright's stories about his introduction to the benefits of iodine and iodine's connection to estriol are both examples of truly spectacular writing. In 1976, from Dr. John Meyers' seminar in Seattle, Wright learned that iodine eliminates the pain of fibrocystic breast disease and often causes rock-like lumps to disappear. Following the Myers' seminar, Wright used iodine in his Tahoma Clinic and helped over one hundred women with fibrocystic breast disease. While tracking an estrogen ratio on these women using a twenty-four-hour urine test (developed by Dr. Henry Lemon at the University of Nebraska), Wright noticed an increase in estriol in all of the women using iodine for their fibrocystic breast disease. And, to think, this is the same hormone that the FDA banned in 2008! There is something terribly wrong with the FDA and something terribly correct with Dr. Jonathan Wright's research!

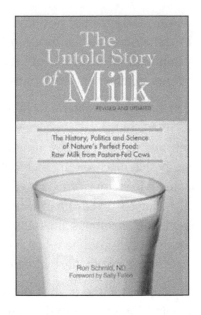

*T*he Untold Story of Milk by Dr. Ron Schmid contains hard-to-obtain information that is well organized and skillfully presented. Readers will feel like they have read several dozen books and articles that are impossible to identify except by a wise few who are awake and paying attention to what has happened in the last sixty to seventy years.

Ron's book is about milk, cows, and the dairy industry, but so much more. Chapter 7, on enzymes, is an example of Ron's gift as a thorough researcher. We're introduced to Dr. Francis Pottenger, who is famous for his cat study that proves the importance of enzyme-rich raw food. I found Dr. Edward Howell's work on enzymes (also covered in chapter 7) particularly interesting due to my own interest in energy medicine. Ron explains that after years of study, Howell became convinced that enzymes must be considered more than simply chemical substances, calling them "matter impregnated with energy values." Howell compares enzymes to batteries that are "possessed of energy" and says:

> *When a battery is "dead," the energy value has vanished; similarly, when enzymes are destroyed by heat, the energy value disappears, leaving behind only a vehicle.*

Ron's thorough presentation covering the work of nutrition pioneer Weston A. Price is particularly evident in a section covering the dairy farmers of Switzerland's Loetschental Valley—a story that serves to clear up modern confusion about fat (a myth created by what Ron calls the medical-industrial complex that says animal fat is bad for us). Price, most known for his book *Nutrition and Physical Degeneration*, was a dentist who lived in Cleveland, Ohio, in the early twentieth century. Due to his interest in teeth, Price and his wife traveled around the world to study the diets of fourteen primitive societies who were free of tooth decay and dental deformities. When Price examined the teeth of children in the Loetschental Valley (an isolated part of the Swiss Alps), he found that those eating unprocessed dairy were nearly free of cavities and all had straight teeth. Young adults who had left the valley experienced tooth decay but showed evidence of remineralization when they returned. Ron tells us that Loetschental dairy samples that Price had analyzed were shown to be far higher in minerals and vitamins than samples of commercial dairy products analyzed from the rest of Europe and North America.

Betrayal by private and public institutions is a story that is told over and over in Ron's book, and each account is equally heartbreaking. Dark clouds have gathered over America in the last century. One glaring example is the malevolent practice of feeding waste grain from distillery operations to dairy cows. Ron explains that early nineteenth century distilleries became dairies when whiskey producers bought cows, fed them slop form their still, and then sold the milk. The slop made cows diseased, led to contaminated milk, and eventually brought compulsory pasteurization laws.

Sadly, Ron reports that the practice of selling leftover grain from alcohol production is *still practiced today*. Land O' Lakes, one of the four multinationals that control 70 percent of the country's fluid milk sales, sells residue from ethanol production to modern confinement dairy operations. Critics in the early nineteenth century called this practice barbaric, and it is equally cruel today. Most people do not realize that the average lifespan of most cows (raised in confinement) is forty-two months, compared to cows on pasture that live twelve to fifteen years.

Ron's book gives us tremendous insights into needed reforms, and for that we are grateful.

CPSIA information can be obtained
at www.ICGtesting.com
Printed in the USA
BVHW091630100222
628615BV00004B/82